American Psychiatry
Past, Present, and Future

American Psychiatry
Past, Present, and Future

Papers presented on the occasion of
the 200th anniversary of the establishment of
the first state-supported mental hospital in America

George Kriegman, M.D., Robert D. Gardner, M.D.,
and D. Wilfred Abse, M.D., Editors

University Press of Virginia
Charlottesville

THE UNIVERSITY PRESS OF VIRGINIA
Copyright © 1975 by the Rector and Visitors
of the University of Virginia

First published 1975

These papers were given at a meeting of
the Southeastern Division of the American
Psychiatric Association. The meeting
was sponsored by the Neuropsychiatric
Society of Virginia, Inc., a District
Branch of the American Psychiatric
Association, and took place October
7–10, 1973, at Williamsburg, Virginia.

Library of Congress Cataloging in Publication Data

American Psychiatric Association. Southeastern
    Division.
    American psychiatry, past, present, and future.

    Includes indexes.
    1. Psychiatry—United States—Congresses.
I. Kriegman, George. II. Gardner, Robert, 1925–
III. Abse, David Wilfred, 1915–   IV. Neuropsy-
chiatric Society of Virginia. V. Title. [DNLM: 1.
Psychiatry—History—United States—Congresses.
WM11 AA1 A5a 1973]   RC443.A7   1975
616.8'9'00973   75-8962   ISBN 0-8139-0571-0

Printed in the United States of America

Contents

The Role of Psychiatry in Society

Preface

THIS book had its origins in 1967 when the American Psychiatric Association approved plans for a divisional meeting to be held in 1973 in Williamsburg, Virginia, to commemorate the founding there, in 1773, of the colonies' first public and state hospital for the mentally ill. The state of Virginia set up a Bicentennial Commission which was originally chaired by Dr. Howard H. Ashbury, Superintendent of Eastern State Hospital. It was Dr. Ashbury's enthusiastic and persistent efforts that led the Neuropsychiatric Society of Virginia to assume the responsibility for the meeting. It is tragic that he died on January 19, 1972, and did not see the realization of his plan. A commemorative plaque in his honor was presented at the opening session of the meeting by the Neuropsychiatric Society of Virginia.

The uniqueness of the occasion—the commemoration of the earliest act of public and state responsibility for the mentally ill in this country—dictated a theme which would appropriately recognize the significance of the occasion and emphasize the continuity of the past with the present. The Program Committee was composed of Drs. William S. Allerton, Robert D. Gardner, Richard W. Garnett, Jr., David R. Hawkins, David B. Kruger, James L. Mathis, Thomas B. Stage, and R. Terrell Wingfield. It was chaired by Dr. George Kriegman.

The committee decided that the usual procedure of inviting papers coordinated with the theme, "American Psychiatry: Past, Present, and Future," would not insure the breadth and depth of discussion that this historic occasion warranted. It was decided, therefore, to invite a group of highly qualified specialists, nonpsychiatric as well as psychiatric, to present papers on specific issues. After considerable deliberation, it was proposed that the first scientific session should give a perspective, the second should be a review of psychiatric therapies, and the third should evaluate the role of psychiatry, and its viability. The committee considered it important to devote one day of the meeting to papers presented primarily by knowledgeable experts outside the field of psychiatry who would critically evaluate the role of psychiatry in the past, the present, and the future. After carefully sifting the long list of eminently qualified psychiatric and nonpsychiatric experts, the committee made its selection, and in 1970 the first invitations went out. The response was most gratifying, and each of the principal speakers had from one to three years' time to prepare his presentation. The profundity of the papers and the ensuing discussions will be evident to the reader.

The editors wish to acknowledge their particular indebtedness and gratitude to Virginia Kennan, Executive Secretary of the Neuropsychiatric Society of Virginia, and Editorial Assistant of the Department of Psychiatry, University of Virginia Medical School. She is to be commended not only for her excellent editorial capabilities but her patience and skill in managing the arrangements that insured the success of the Williamsburg meeting, for which Barbara Garland, the past Executive Secretary of the Society, did so much to prepare. We are also heavily indebted to Kay B. Sneed, who undertook the arduous secretarial task of transcribing the audiotapes of the discussions that followed the scientific presentations.

Acknowledgments are also made to the following firms and agencies which insured the financial success of the Williamsburg meeting by their support of the scientific programs and/or their participation as exhibitors: Abbott Laboratories, Dictaphone Corporation, Edgemeade, Geigy Pharmaceuticals, Hoffmann La Roche, Inc., Lakeside Laboratories, Inc., Merck, Sharp & Dohme, McNeil Laboratories, Pennwalt Corporation, Pfizer, Inc., Psychiatric Institutes of America, Inc., A. H. Robins Co., Roerig, St. Elizabeth's Hospital, Sandoz Pharmaceuticals, Smith Kline & French Laboratories, the South Carolina Department of Mental Health, E. R. Squibb & Sons, Inc., and the Veterans Administration.

GEORGE KRIEGMAN, M.D.
ROBERT D. GARDNER, M.D.
D. WILFRED ABSE, M.D.

Introduction

George Kriegman, M.D.
D. Wilfred Abse, M.D.

THE 200th anniversary of the establishment of North America's first public mental hospital is a propitious occasion and an appropriate moment for us to consider where psychiatry has been, where it is at present, and where it is going.

As physicians, we have long recognized that in arriving at a diagnosis a thorough knowledge of the patient's past medical history is as important as the physical examination and subsequent laboratory procedures. Similarly, we have realized that although prognostic evaluations are required, caution must be exercised in predicting the eventual consequences of our therapeutic endeavors. In this series of papers and the ensuing discussions an attempt has been made to examine the field of psychiatry in the same reflective, analytic fashion that we use in evaluating an individual patient.

It has long been a truism in medicine that it is inadvisable for a physician to attend to his own ailments and that subjective feelings may interfere with objective evaluation of the disease. In organizing the commemorative meeting at which these papers were first presented, it was recognized that knowledgeable experts outside the clinical practice of psychiatry are important in validating our evaluations and in suggesting any remedies we need to consider.

Interestingly, the psychiatrist acknowledges, in the papers and discussions recorded here, challenges to his usual professional identity. These challenges reflect not only scientific progress but societal alterations of considerable magnitude. Convergent and divergent views are expressed. In accordance with the occasion these thought-provoking contributions are infused with the drama of two centuries of psychiatric endeavor.

As the official spokesman for the American Psychiatric Association, Dr. John Spiegel opened the conference with a "laundry list" of administrative concerns that vex psychiatrists today, and recommended attention to their moral dimensions. In reviewing six models with which a psychiatrist might identify he asked that the implications of each be pondered and their inconsistencies reduced—or at least that each be assigned a place in a soberly evaluated hierarchy of importance. His remarks acknowledge the possibility, all too apparent in our "enlightened" society, that any endeavor born in compassionate concern for human suffering can, almost imperceptibly, become the "cause" of a self-serving and self-protective professional community that has mislaid its original commitment.

Dr. Norman Dain, the authoritative historian of American psychiatry of the 18th century, challenges the ahistorical and the linear progressive view of the history of psychiatry. "In evaluating the past one cannot and should not forget the present, but at the same time it is misleading to judge past phenomena without reference to their own historical context. Nor can it be assumed that later is better—that psychiatry has evolved in a linear, upward direction." Dr. Dain carefully traces the management of the mentally ill from the home care stage with its primary emphasis on folk remedies, religious rites, and custodial care in the 1700s through the post-Revolutionary period of the establishment of mental hospitals with the enlightened recognition that mental disorders were natural diseases, not demonic states, and that they were potentially curable. Dr. Dain also outlines the unique role of the Eastern State Hospital at Williamsburg, Virginia, and of the Galt family. He completes his historical account with a detailed description of the rise and fall of moral treatment.

Dr. John Romano, the distinguished psychiatric scholar and educator, lists in his Keynote Address 15 significant and important contributions, achievements, and trends in American psychiatry. He outlines the growth in the field of psychiatry, the number of psychiatric practitioners, and the role of psychiatry in medicine, particularly in the last 25 years. He delineates the two major theories that influence psychiatry—the psychosocial theory stemming from the work of Sigmund Freud, and the genetic biological theory—and discusses their polarization. He foresees a return, in what remains of this century, to emphasis on the care and treatment of persons suffering from psychosis, addiction, alcoholism, chronic mental disorder, and old age. Dr. Romano urges that the psychiatrist of the future consider himself first and foremost a clinician in spite of the identity confusion he is likely to experience as his task undergoes further definition.

With these perspectives furnishing a broad framework, the papers in the following section specifically examine three major therapeutic orientations. Dr. James L. Mathis, in his introduction to this section, "Mainstreams of Therapeutic Modalities," sustains the proper historical attitude with a brief, to-the-point review. He concludes with the "hope that our followers will acknowledge that their improvements will be built upon the painfully laid foundations of the past, however primitive and crude they may appear to them in retrospect."

Dr. Lawrence Kolb, the distinguished educator, administrator, and psychoanalyst, dissects the evolution of psychological approaches in the treatment of the mentally ill from the time of Chiarugi to the introduction of Freud's psychodynamic principles. He cites the significant roles played by Adolf Meyer and William A. White, and the contributions of Brill, Dunbar, Schilder, Healy, Alexander, and Sullivan. He comments on the ready reception psychoanalytic concepts had in a country in which men from many lands were drawing together in social experimentation in a still evolving nation. Giving a comprehensive overview of the many tributaries of special interest that flow into the mainstream of American psychiatry—particularly group and family therapy—Dr. Kolb declares that the psychotherapist of today has the breadth of knowledge and theory and the technical capability to effect a useful combination of psychotherapy and somatic treatment.

It has been said that man uses both the practical arts and the applied sciences. In the latter he applies ascertained principles to particular cases, but a practical art like medical healing—and this includes psychiatry—has no complete and sure foundation of ascertained principles in spite of the vast experience that lies behind its rules. These rules are not to be rigidly applied in any given case since they fall short of being scientific principles, but are to be interpreted by clinical judgment and intuition. It might be well to warn some of the dissident factions in psychiatry that when the measurements of success appropriate for an applied science are adapted for use with a practical art they may be no longer instruments for improvement but tools for the justification of quackery. Certainly the psychiatrist's practice of psychotherapy remains to a large extent an art in spite of its increasing validation in science, so it is not surprising that divergent views appear in these pages. We may be less likely to yield to "fallacious pressure" after a study of these thought-provoking contributions, infused as they are with the drama of two centuries of patient search for mental wholeness, and newly aware that prejudice and a certain sophisticated insularity may account for some of our vociferous but often short-lived enthusiasms about both theory and practice.

Dr. Seymour Kety, whose brilliant biological research into psychiatric disorders is widely recognized, analyzes the progress made in understanding the biological factors in psychiatric disorders, with particular emphasis on the major problem of schizophrenia. He outlines the two current hypotheses regarding the etiology of schizophrenia: the transmethylation hypothesis and the central catecholamine synapses hypothesis. He highlights the central and special role of dopamine in the treatment of this disorder, and its relationship to the phenothiazines, the butyrophenones, and the tricyclic antidepressants. In regard to a biological explanation of schizophrenia Dr. Kety declares that "we are beginning to see the light at the end of the tunnel."

Dr. Melvin Sabshin, distinguished psychiatric educator, administrator, and writer, reminds us in his comprehensive discussion of social-community approaches in psychiatry that the American Revolution and its sequelae initiated many humanitarian movements, the moral treatment movement among them. Dr. Sabshin defines social psychiatry as the use of *"independent* social variables to predict and to explain a series of *dependent* psychiatric variables" and the involvement of "the rational employment of *independent* social variables . . . to alter *dependent* psychiatric variables." He goes on to discuss the three major sectors of social psychiatry: the geographic, organizational, or spatial; the developmental systems in which age-specific adaptation is required; and functional therapeutic processes. He laments the relative decline of social psychiatry at the present time, and recognizes that it has come about largely because of the shift to the community psychiatry approach. Although supportive of this move, he points out that the higher priority it gives to pragmatic solutions compared with its attention to scientific issues threatens the accountability of community psychiatry. He optimistically anticipates that we will "find a blend of that enlightened humanism which glowed so warmly in the era of moral treatment with the scientific positivism and transactional system approaches of this century."

The discussion that followed the presentations of Drs. Kolb, Kety, and Sabshin adds further dimensions to their papers and contains much that is thought-provoking.

The next section of this book deals with the broader philosophical question of the nature and appropriateness of the role of psychiatry in the present and in the future. In introducing this section Dr. David R. Hawkins mourns the loss of an earlier confidence in an inevitably brighter day to come, and the pervasive uncertainty about psychiatry's proper function in our time. He acknowledges the interface of social science and psychiatry, and asks how the social scientist views psychiatry's role.

Dr. Charles Rosenberg, as a historian, questions "psychiatry's social legitimacy." He points to three areas in which psychiatry is under special pressure; in its relationship to society and its needs; in its relationship to medicine; and in the divisions within its own house. Examining these in detail, he concludes that psychiatry is facing a legitimacy crisis and that it must justify its role as a specialty among the healing arts.

Dr. Morris Schwartz, who is an eminent sociologist, emphasizes the reciprocal interplay of society and psychiatry, focusing on the phenomenon of de-humanization, which he regards as a destructive force with which psychiatry is directly concerned. He identifies six forms: psychosocial reduction; status immersion; routinization; de-personing; object-making; and reification. He challenges the profession to make a value choice—either to maintain a "neutral" stance (which he views as one of self-deception) or to take an active part in opposing de-humanization. He urges that "psychiatry . . . join with others to constitute a pressure group opposing de-humanizing societal processes and encouraging institutional humanization."

Judge David Bazelon, the distinguished jurist, addresses himself to the problem of the psychiatrist's accountability. He attacks the self-protective, equivocal stance of psychiatry, and its reluctance to submit its professional judgments to public review. Judge Bazelon feels that psychiatry "has generated much of the current crisis of confidence which is rapidly undermining public trust." Noting sadly that psychiatrists fail to understand the adversary process, he outlines its essential features and calls on the profession to undertake "a kind of *self*-analysis to ensure that its power rests on its expertise rather than its prestige."

Dr. Roy Grinker, Sr., a renowned psychiatrist and psychoanalyst, concludes this discussion of psychiatry's role in society, and its viability. Integrating the relevant social and cultural factors, he gives a comprehensive review of the various roles and types of psychiatry and delineates the "multiple psychiatries"—the psychotherapists, the somatotherapists, and the sociotherapists. Turning to society's loss of faith in psychiatry, and the present climate of anti-intellectualism, he scolds the profession for its participation in the general return to mysticism. Dr. Grinker calls for a systems approach to psychiatry and defines psychiatry as a biopsychosocial system that should be able to develop a unified theory of human behavior.

The second discussion period further clarifies and expands the points raised by each of the speakers. Dr. Kramer's paper on demographic factors of the present and those anticipated for the future as problems for psychiatry forms a fitting appendix to this long view of American psychiatry. Subject to future social and political philosophies, the growing need for more mental health services and more personnel that seems to loom ahead emphasizes the urgency that the profession establish its priorities.

The major theme of these papers and the discussions that followed their presentation is the humanistic but triphasic spiral course that American psychiatry has followed over the last 200 years. Each of the three major fields of psychiatry—the psychological, the biological, and the social—has become increasingly differentiated from the other, and hierarchically organized to the point at which each claims the body of psychiatry for its own. Such separation has led to the conceptual distancing and alienation that has precipitated the present crisis of credibility for psychiatry today. Rivalrous proprietary contentions have led society to demand that our profession validate its legitimacy, credibility, and accountability. Understandably, the secondary theme repeatedly surfacing in these papers is the imperative need to reconcile, coalesce, and integrate the three fields into a unified theory of human behavior and a unified approach to its therapy. In any event, partitive approaches that masquerade as comprehensive systems can obviously be misleading.

American Psychiatry
Past, Present, and Future

1. *Opening Remarks*

Robert D. Gardner, M.D.

THERE is inescapable drama in considering in Colonial Williamsburg our efforts to ameliorate the human state in the 1970s. The establishment of the first mental hospital in the colonies, in a Virginia newly claimed from the wilderness and still pastoral, is remote in time, and incredibly remote in ambience. But it is difficult in this environment to escape a feeling of compelling identification with those early Virginians, and a sobering sense of having inherited a kind of trust.

I should like to open this program with a dedication. While preparing for this dedication I pondered the question: To whom would it be fitting and proper to dedicate such a convocation? For guidance I looked to our theme, "American Psychiatry: Past, Present, and Future," and wondered who from the past was the leader in treating the insane, the feebleminded, the mentally incompetent. Should it be Dr. Benjamin Rush, "the Father of American Psychiatry," a signer of the Declaration of Independence? Or should it be Governor Fauquier of Virginia, who, in 1769, pressed the colonial Virginia Assembly to provide a public hospital for the treatment of the mentally ill? Or Dr. John Minson Galt, first superintendent of Eastern Lunatic Asylum, and one of Virginia's two founders of the American Psychiatric Association's original thirteen? Or should it be Dr. Howard Ashbury, the late superintendent of Eastern State Hospital, who was dedicated, respected by staff and patients, and devoted to Eastern State Hospital and the Bicentennial that had been so many years in the planning? Should it be one of our distinguished speakers from the present, or some other great leader in American psychiatry? Or can one predict a future psychiatric revolution that deserves our tribute?

Any one of these seemed proper, but somehow none seemed quite fitting. And then my deliberation focused on an obvious selection: we must dedicate our proceedings to American *patients,* past, present, and future. That is our oath, our commandment, our trust. For 200 years it is *they* who have tolerated *our* insanity, *our* feeblemindedness, and *our* mental incompetence!

2. *The Bicentennial of Eastern State Hospital*

Robert D. Gardner, M.D.

I N PRECISELY the same month that Philippe Pinel of France was
graduated in medicine at the University of Toulouse and
20 years before his celebrated unchaining of the mentally ill at
the Salpêtrière, a milestone in the history of American psychiatry
took place. On October 12, 1773, a psychotic Virginian was taken
from the jail in Williamsburg, where he had lain for almost eight
months, and was escorted across town to more suitable quarters.
He had committed no crime, but had been thought dangerous
and held in jail because there had been no other place to keep
people like him who were "ideots" or "lunaticks." The new
brick building on Francis Street, later to be known as Eastern
State Hospital, had been built by the Virginia Colony as a "public hospital for persons of insane and disordered minds." The
admission of that patient signaled the opening of not only the
first publicly supported hospital for the care of the mentally ill
in North America but also the first devoted exclusively to the
treatment of mental patients. (Earlier, in 1752, the Pennsylvania
Hospital in Philadelphia, which had accommodations for mental
patients, had been established as the first private general hospital
in the colonies.)

In Virginia, until the public hospital in Williamsburg was
opened, mentally disordered persons who had families to care for
them were kept confined to one room of their homes. Such was
the fate of the first wife of Patrick Henry. Less fortunate insane
paupers were cared for—when they were cared for at all—by the
vestries of the parishes in which they lived. Care was limited to
those who were considered violent or dangerous, and consisted of
either confinement in jail or in privately built log cages. Those
considered harmless and peaceful were neglected or abused and
left to wander, unkempt, in rags and often starving.

They were not completely unnoticed, however. In 1766, Governor Francis Fauquier, the son of a French physician and a man

generally sympathetic to the needs of his people in the Virginia Colony, attempted to educate the colonists concerning their responsibility for the mentally ill. In an eloquent speech to the Virginia General Assembly he made a stirring appeal to their "consideration and humanity," recommending the establishment of a public hospital for the care of "those unfortunate individuals who are so unhappy as to be deprived of their reason." A resolution by the House of Burgesses endorsed his proposal, but it was referred to a committee. Nothing was done until 1770, two years after Fauquier's death, when, during the administration of his successor, the popular Lord Botetourt, Fauquier's recommendation was enacted into law. Under its provision a "Court of Directors" was appointed to supervise the construction of the hospital and to administer its affairs thereafter. The bill made an appropriation to cover the initial capital outlay for the building, and outlined commitment and discharge procedures.

Thus the hospital was founded on the principle that the public was responsible for providing care for those who needed it, whether they were able to pay or not. (Those who could pay were charged 15 pounds of tobacco per year.) Not only was hospital care provided, but also transportation to Williamsburg from the outlying areas; the first patient was from Hanover County. This meant that sheriffs throughout the Commonwealth who had been detaining mentally disordered individuals now had an incentive to take them to the Williamsburg hospital for more appropriate care. Thus, in 1773, seven years after Fauquier's initial appeal to the good conscience of the community, it came to pass that Virginia not only recognized the needs of the mentally ill but publicly supported the delivery of a service system. Virginians passed enabling statutes, established a pioneering department of mental health, and promoted a concept of treatment intervention rather than incarceration alone. Interestingly, the establishment by law of the first public mental hospital came before Virginia had free public schools or even freedom from England.

Under the provisions of the law 15 public-spirited citizens were given lifetime appointments to the Court of Directors. The first membership roster reads like a "Who's Who" of colonial Williamsburg. Among those named were such distinguished Virginians as Peyton Randolph, speaker of the House of Burgesses; George Wythe, clerk of that same body; Thomas Nelson, secretary of the colony; John Blair; John Blair, Jr.; Robert Carter; John Tazewell; Thomas Everard; and Robert Carter Nicholas.

The original hospital was a two-story rectangular building 100 by 32 feet in size. The first floor had 12 patient rooms and an apartment for the "keeper." The second floor had another 12 rooms for patients and a meeting room for the Court of Directors, which in an emergency could be divided into two rooms for patients.

The Court of Directors met weekly and considered each application for admission. Some applicants were turned away as incurable. Thirty-six patients were admitted the first year.

James Galt of Williamsburg, who was not a physician, was appointed the first keeper. He was empowered to call in Dr. John deSequeyra to see each patient on his first admission and thereafter whenever necessary. Thus Dr. deSequeyra became the first visiting physician to the hospital.

Little is known as to what treatment was given to the first patients. At the time, Benjamin Rush of Philadelphia, now known as "the Father of American Psychiatry," was four years out of medical school and was prescribing purging and puking, blisters and clysters. Believing that insanity was due to congestion of blood in the brain, he frequently performed phlebotomy. Although not an advocate of restraint by incarceration, he did use a restraining chair known as "the tranquilizer," which he felt was more therapeutic than a straitjacket, and which made it easier to administer purgatives and phlebotomy when necessary.

During the Revolution operation of the hospital was suspended due to lack of funds, and the building was used to quarter troops. It was reopened in 1783 and has been in continuous operation since. James Galt—by then a war veteran—resumed his post as keeper. The name Galt was to be integrally involved with Eastern State Hospital. When James Galt died in 1800 he was succeeded by William T. Galt, who served until his death in 1826. Subsequently, a number of keepers succeeded him until 1841, when Dr. John Minson Galt II was appointed superintendent by an act of the Virginia Assembly, which now required that the head of the hospital be a physician. Dr. Alexander D. Galt and Dr.

John Minson Galt, Dr. Galt's father and grandfather, respectively, had served as visiting physicians (but not superintendents) before him.

At the time of the election of Dr. John M. Galt II to be first superintendent there were 125 patients at the hospital. It had had a steady growth from 1800, and an investigating committee reported serious overcrowding and suggested that another hospital be erected in the western part of the state. Thus, in 1828 Western State Hospital was established at Staunton. During the 1800s, as the population grew and as new or different forms of treatment were added to the hospitals' armamentarium, more land and facilities were acquired to provide such care. Dr. Galt instituted programs of "moral treatment" which included occupational, recreational, musical, and industrial therapy. He saw to it that the library was well stocked, that musical instruments were available, and that occupational and craft shops were provided. There were regular classes of instruction, and patients could earn academic certification. Recreational programs included games, carriage rides, and entertainments by visiting bands who came to play at the hospital. Dr. Galt appointed a full-time chaplain to the hospital. He boarded many of the patients with residents of Williamsburg, using what we may now regard as an early example of foster home care or halfway house placement. He invited the ladies of Williamsburg to visit the patients and do whatever they could for them. This was the beginnings of the hospital's volunteer services.

Galt recognized the need of classification and placement of patients according to their needs and status. He often separated the acutely ill from the chronic patients. He had graduated from the University of Pennsylvania and was proficient in European languages. His textbook, *The Treatment of Insanity,** was a widely known and authoritative compendium of then current knowledge gleaned from publications throughout Europe and America. He differed with his predecessors in deploring the extensive use of bloodletting and in favoring the "moral treatment" described above.

Dr. Galt was an avid correspondent and kept in touch with superintendents of all the well-known state and psychiatric hos-

* Published in 1846 by Harper & Brothers, N.Y. Reprinted in 1973 by Arno Press, N.Y.

pitals of that era. He was one of the 13 founders of the Association of Medical Superintendents in 1844. This later became the American Psychiatric Association.

Dr. Galt's tenure at the hospital continued until 1862. His reign came to a sudden and dramatic end during the Civil War, when, after the battle of Williamsburg, the hospital was occupied by Union troops and Dr. Galt was barred from entering its grounds. He died 12 days later of a heart attack.

Although Federal troops continued their occupation of Williamsburg and the hospital for the rest of the war, the institution continued to be used exclusively for the care of the mentally ill, whether military or civilian, from both North and South. The hospital was returned to the state of Virginia on October 28, 1865.

After the Civil War the hospital entered a period of marked growth which continued for the next 100 years. It was not until 1894 that it received its present name of Eastern State Hospital. There have been 13 superintendents, all physicians, since the Civil War. The original buildings are no longer in existence due to a series of fires. The original site is now a grassy plot within the boundaries of the Colonial Williamsburg restoration. Colonial Williamsburg, Inc., has plans to reconstruct an exact copy of the first building on its original foundations. The modern Eastern State Hospital has been transplanted to a location about three miles from the older site.

As a fitting tribute to the pioneering spirit, ideas, and conditions intertwined with the history of Virginia's Eastern State Hospital, the American Psychiatric Association and its local district branch, the Neuropsychiatric Society of Virginia, commemorated the bicentennial by holding its Southeastern Divisional Meeting in Williamsburg on October 7–10, 1973. The theme of the meeting held on the occasion of the historic celebration in Williamsburg was, appropriately, "American Psychiatry: Past, Present and Future." The presentation generated such interest that it was decided to publish the proceedings, as we have done on these pages.

The good Governor Fauquier, asleep under the floor of Bruton Parish Church, can rest assured not only that his dream was fulfilled but that his institution served as a model for the nation — and is carrying its influence forward into its third century.

3. Conflicts in Ideologies and Values

John P. Spiegel, M.D., President of the American Psychiatric Association

I BRING you greetings from Dr. Alfred Freedman, president of the American Psychiatric Association, who was originally scheduled to make this presentation. He is unable to be here because he is in Russia attending the meeting of the International Psychiatric Association; the content of my message should be "from Russia with love," except that I am not sure how much love there is in situ in view of some of the current problems, the differences in attitudes in the USSR and the United States about the Israeli war, to say nothing of the issue raised by the American Psychiatric Association shortly before Dr. Freedman and others left to attend the meeting—the issue of the misuse (or abuse) of psychiatry in Russia to deal with political dissent. I do not know if you are aware of the position taken by the American Psychiatric Association that the question of the possible misuse of psychiatry in Russia can no longer be ignored; members of our Association who are there now are presumably engaged in at least raising that question with our Russian colleagues.

It has been traditional at this sort of meeting for the newly elected officers of the American Psychiatric Association to talk about what is new in the APA, what is going on, from the point of view of the Board, and so on. I thought I would depart somewhat from that tradition and use the short time available to me to review with you some of the problems and conflicts in the profession of psychiatry, trying to get down to some of the basic controversies that really trouble us in our everyday life and that are continually brought to the attention of the officers of the APA.

I suppose to conform, to gear into the theme of this meeting, I should call my talk "Past, Present, and Future Problems and Conflicts of the Profession," and I will touch on the time element in reviewing the subject; but what I actually intend to do is to begin with a list of the problems confronting us so that we may have some concrete account of present difficulties and issues—and then spend most of my time trying to present my view of the conflicts of values and ideology that underlie them, regarding the problems themselves as symptoms or that relatively small part of the iceberg that is visible. I feel that unless we understand the underlying value problems and conflicts in their historical focus we are going to have great difficulty resolving the particular problems that we face. I hope no one will feel that I am limiting my talk to the difficulties and weaknesses of our profession, or accenting them unduly without appreciation of the positive achievements of American psychiatry, which are enormous. But right now—at this moment in time, as they say in Washington—I think it highly important that we look at our problems:

Now, to list them: There are problems involving third-party insurance carriers. I should say that each of these problems has something good and something bad about it—which is why they are matters of controversy. We know that one of the things that will happen where third-party insurance is concerned—which is already happening in connection with private carriers and which will probably be more marked if there is government health insurance—is the amplification of facilities to care for increasing numbers of the patient population in our country. The positive gain here is unlikely to come about, however, without enormous interference occasioned by this sort of overview and the insertion of an outside force into our ordinary relations with our patients. The problem must eventually be resolved.

Secondly, associated with the problem of third-party carriers is that of confidentiality. It is not necessary to discuss these problems in any detail because we are all familiar with them. I merely want to say that the problem of confidentiality, which is very great and increasing daily with third-party carriers, is complicated on the one hand by demands for information about the patient, particularly in computerized systems, with all the evil effects that might characterize such systems eventually in terms of the correlation and pooling of information into computerized systems. But on the other hand, providing such information to computers, with their large-scale capacity to survey what is going on with respect to treatment, can be seen as justified by the resultant availability of adequate information about treatment problems. The problem of confidentiality will continue to trouble us; it certainly has not been made any simpler by issues ventilated be-

fore the Watergate Committee. Everyone knows how easy it is to
get information about a patient. All private lawyers in this room
know how easy it is to get information about any patient; all you
have to do is to get in touch with some nurse, some doctor, or
some paraprofessional. As if that were not an ethical problem.

Another one of the problems is the accountability associated
with the third-party carrier and amplification of insurance programs. Accountability has many different components. Certainly
if outside carriers are going to pay for care one can understand
their need to have an account of what it is they are paying for.
But accountability raises the problem of peer review and interference with the normal practice and relations between doctors
and patients. It raises the issue of continuing education and re-
certification with some of the phoniness likely to accompany this
effort to have everyone prove in some way that he has kept his
medical and psychiatric skills up to date; and there is also the
problem of citizen (consumer) input, which can disrupt normal
doctor-patient relationships. Nevertheless, on the positive side
one can understand and perhaps appreciate increased public interest in the kind of care being provided.

Another problem has to do with the hospitalization of patients
with serious mental illness, and with associated right-to-treatment
suits. There is the impact of the whole legal apparatus on medical
care, particularly in hospitals. Another difficulty arises from tension between private practice and other types of service care
systems, including community mental health, which are alter-
nating and shifting health care into directions entirely new to us,
directions for which we are in some respects ill prepared, and
which at times seem disorderly. Another problem has to do with
manpower recruitment and training—not only the government
cutbacks that make it difficult to recruit and train psychiatric
residents, but related difficulties such as the shortage of doctors,
the increasing use of foreign medical school graduates in supple-
menting care in psychiatric hospitals, the concentration of psychiatrists in particular urban areas, and so forth. There is also
tension between the medical practice situation for which we are
trained and the administrative situations to which many of us are
being introduced. It is becoming increasingly important for our
profession to engage in policy-making, administrative planning,

and the implementation of programs, activities roughly included under the rubric of administrative psychiatry but for which we have not had training although the public demands it of us.

I have given an incomplete list. I could talk about psychosurgery, behavior modification, and other procedures which, particularly as they concern inmates in our maximum security institutions, are now becoming highly controversial. I could talk about the public's loss of confidence in the profession of psychiatry as a whole, the deterioration of our image, so to speak. I am not going to try to extend my list, but I want to have some concrete matters before us in order to discuss what I think is perhaps more important—What are the ideological and value conflicts that underlie these current problems that beset our profession? A review of the list—any particular item in it or all of them together—reveals, I think, that each has two sides. In one way or another the questions are being asked, Are we meeting our moral responsibility where patient care is concerned? Are we really meeting the need? Are we attentive to ethical issues or merely considering our own professional vested self-interest? Such moral or ethical questions can be dealt with more easily, I think, if one looks at the conflicts and the troubles in our profession against a background of historical evolution.

This is where I want to introduce the time element. I think it is easier to deal with those conflicts in terms of six models of professional psychiatric practice which have evolved over time in the background of what we do. The first is the "priest magician" model—the shaman, the omniscient and omnipotent faith healer model, which, I am sure, no member of our profession officially accepts nowadays. This role might be assigned to us by some members of the public. It seems to some that we are sitting with our X-ray eyes, eager to jump on others and analyze them and so forth. So there remain ways, however informally sanctioned, in which the faith healer image still troubles us—and one that we have to be very careful to deal with.

The second model is the medical model. Rather than speak in terms of the usual clichés I should like to discuss it in context of an article by Erving Goffman with which you may not be familiar. Goffman gave his paper the intriguing title, "The Medical Model of Mental Hospitalization, Some Notes on the Vicissitudes of the

Tinkering Trade."* A provocative sociologist, Goffman discusses medical practice from the point of view of all tinkers; that is to say, he compares it with the model of the radio repairman and the automobile mechanic. Although the doctor is in all respects at the top of an elite hierarchy of tinkers (and psychiatrists are certainly near the peak of prestige within this) the whole tinkering model has common elements. Goffman discusses them with some hyperbole. Indeed, I also use hyperbole throughout my discussion of models, exaggerating to emphasize certain points. Goffman says that this model is like that of any automobile mechanic or radio or TV repairman; the owner brings the object in for repair or maintenance, and the tinker looks at it and makes a diagnosis. Then he tells what's wrong, what you have to do, how much it will cost, and how long it will take to get it fixed. He makes all these determinations with an impersonal attitude. Inasmuch as the transaction is one between the owner of the object and the tinker, medical practice itself has many of these same impersonal and mechanistic elements, the difference being, of course, that you cannot trade in your psyche. It is not easy, in fact, to trade in your body, but you can get new tubes and aortas and things like that. The mental apparatus, however, cannot very well be replaced, although I often think one of the problems with psychosurgery is tinkering. Something up there in the brain is going to be taken out, something substituted, or put in, and perhaps the personality will be modified in some significant way. At any rate, good and bad elements conflict in the tinkering model, which I will discuss no further since I just want to open it up for future dialogue.

The third of these models is the missionary model, all the way from Dorothea Dix through the mental hygiene movement and the mental health movement; it is an ameliorative model. Practice in our profession is charged with helping people, people with very serious human difficulties; with removing stigma; with making life easier for the suffering—a humanistic outlook in contrast to the mechanistic outlook of the tinkering models. This model is not without problems itself, especially in its extreme interpretation that the humanitarian impulse can make one successful in taking care of almost anything; that there is a mental

* *Asylums: Essays on the Social Situation of Mental Patients and Other Inmates* (New York: Doubleday, 1961).

health solution to any human experience, including war. Such a view makes for exaggerated optimism.

The fourth is the industrial model or the industrial-commercial model. The term "the health services industry," is commonly used now. In many ways what we are coming to do can be compared to the commercial-industrial model. We make a product, so to speak, but just as Ford products range from the Lincoln Continental to the Pinto, so we have a range from high-class psychoanalysts—Park Avenue or Hollywood types for those who can afford them—to mental health personnel in the storefront facility, the outreach clinic, and so forth. There are different varieties of mental health care for different socioeconomic levels. This diverse product is brought to the consumer by a variety of middlemen; it has to be packaged in different ways with appropriate labels, and like the industrial-commercial products, it has a certain amount of obsolescence in it. Some therapies go out of style as new therapies come in. I recently read about one called "tickle therapy," described, as best I can recall, in *Time* magazine. At any rate, the packaging, distribution, and so forth are closely modeled on the industrial-commercial distribution system and the Better Business aspects of any such model. This is where the consumer comes in, because if there is to be a variety of packaging with a variety of prices and a diversity of products, certainly the consumer wants to know whether he is getting what he is paying for, and some people will be engaged in protecting the consumer's interest.

The fifth model is the scientific model, which I will not elaborate for lack of time; but we do attempt to establish our profession on the basis of the most vigorous aspects of scientific research, plowing back the results of that research into either the tinkering model or the industrial service–distribution model. A problem with the scientific research model is that it comes close to the hustle that characterizes industrial research for profit. One has to know where to go with one's research project, one has to have lines of connection with appropriate powers in government, and so forth, in order to get the funding to do the research. One has even sometimes to adapt one's research to funding provisions, making certain to do something that is popular enough to be funded, perhaps at the expense of a master interest without wide appeal. Moral and ethical issues are again involved.

And, lastly, there is the political model, with its prospect of putting our profession into areas upon the threshold of which we find ourselves already. This involves lobbying at local, state, and federal levels in order to influence the government to provide the kinds of resources our work requires. Much more could be said about all of these things. I have just wanted to open up discussion about them and to end with emphasis on the fact that I see serious conflicts among the models and within each of them taken singly. What confronts the profession is the need to integrate these diverse models as they have evolved. There they are. They need to be articulated; they need to be analyzed; they need to be discussed; and they need to be resolved. We need to resolve the conflicts rather than to behave defensively as we so often do. Instead of saying, "How can you say that about psychiatrists?" I think what we have to do is to roll up our sleeves and get to work to integrate the models and to resolve the conflicts. If we cannot resolve them we can at least draw up a set of priorities on the basis of importance. I am not going to try to present you with my own personal priorities or my solution to these various problems because that is not my role here this morning. But I thought it would be helpful, especially in view of the presentations that will be made from the point of view of the history of our profession, simply to open up these matters for you.

4. American Psychiatry in the 18th Century

Norman Dain, PH.D.

THERE is a tendency today to view the history of psychiatry ahistorically, particularly in reference to mental hospitals; that is, to condemn early workers in the mental health field for not operating from the perspectives of the present. According to one historian, for example, the fact that mental hospitals could evolve into snake pits shows that an as institution the mental hospital in the United States did not at its inception represent a step forward in the treatment of mental disorder; that it had from the very beginning inherent defects that made inevitable its deterioration into something grimly custodial. It never even promised to be "a rose garden."

Because the community health approach is in vogue today it is concluded that the mentally disordered should never have been removed from the community in the first place, that mental hospitals never were a positive force. This position does not essentially differ from the Aristotelian argument that the conclusion of an act is inherent in its inception, but when cause and effect are separated by decades—even a century or two—one may be pardoned for regarding this argument with skepticism. Moreover, the assumption that the condemnation applies to all mental hospitals is unwarranted; not all became snake pits, however little they may have offered their inmates by way of "cure."

An older and more widespread attitude distorts the past in a different way. The further one looks back in history, it posits, the more inadequate the treatment of mental patients was. This viewpoint is sustained by more than the belief in progress traditional in the Western world, particularly in America. It gains credence also from the assumption that science is a cumulative process, that since psychiatry is a part of science, psychiatric knowledge and practice at any given time therefore surpass what was previously available. The advances of medicine in the modern scientific era support this view.

I would like to challenge both these positions with respect to the psychiatry of the 18th and early 19th century in the United States. In evaluating the past one cannot and should not forget the present, but at the same time it is misleading to judge past phenomena without reference to their own historical context. Nor can it be assumed that later is better—that psychiatry has evolved in a linear, upward direction.

The first mental hospitals in British North America, opened during the middle and at the end of the 18th century, were, I believe, therapeutic in intent and, to a modest degree, in practice. They were designed to meet realistic problems posed by mentally disordered persons living under urban conditions, and were inspired by humanitarian impulses, however elitist and paternalistic. With increasing density of population, family care proved inadequate—if, indeed, it ever had been satisfactory in the smaller communities of the 17th and early 18th centuries—and some people recognized the need for a systematic humane way of dealing with the mentally disordered. Placement in jails and almshouses was rejected as a solution because the leaders of colonial and then post-Revolutionary American society adopted toward human ills the hopeful attitudes associated with the Enlightenment. They regarded mental disorders as natural diseases, not as invasions of the devil or divine retribution for sin, and looked to hospitals as refuges for the unhappy victims in which they could be made well again. Other motives were the desire to protect society from possible harm from so-called maniacs and to relieve families of the burden of care. The optimistic spirit of 18th-century Americans was not, however, matched by an effective therapeutic system; the psychiatry of that time could be only marginally therapeutic, like medicine in general. It was later, beginning in the 1790s, that a new therapy was introduced; it flourished for some 50 years, and at its best it far surpassed in quality the care given mental patients before and afterward until well into our own time.

Our knowledge about mental disorders in the 18th century, especially in its first half, is quite limited. Most persons considered dangerous or sufficiently bothersome to require some form of restraint were probably kept at home. Communities sometimes subsidized a poor family to keep one of its members under control, or paid strangers to perform this function. A small propor-

tion of so-called insane or violent or physically handicapped "lunatics" who could not be kept at home were incarcerated in the jails and almshouses built by large towns and cities, and an indeterminate number of such people wandered freely through the towns and around the countryside. They were seldom treated by physicians.

We know little about how families dealt with their patients, partly because of the secrecy surrounding mental disorder, and also because of the absence of authentic case histories. Although historians report terrible examples of mistreatment, there is not enough evidence to conclude that insane persons in family care were, in fact, ordinarily neglected or mistreated. Nevertheless, if the information we do have is any guide, the mentally ill did not fare very well at home. People so dependent on others usually pay a high price for whatever care they receive, even from their closest relations, and this was no doubt especially true in the past, when laymen commonly held the mentally ill morally responsible for their condition. Considering the paucity of physicians and the low state of medicine at the time, few patients at home could have received medical attention; folk remedies and religious rites to drive out evil spirits were probably more common. Certainly from the community's standpoint the purpose of home care was custodial rather than therapeutic; it was not seen as offering a good prospect for recovery but as a convenient shelter and a way to protect the community. Indeed, in England the private madhouses of the 18th century grew out of the practice of boarding out the insane in homes.

By the middle of the century a new alternative, the urban hospital, appeared in the colonies. Although state mental hospitals today tend to be remote from centers of population and are criticized on that account, they were not always so located. The first hospitals stood in or near the capital cities of the colonies (later to become states) —Philadelphia, Williamsburg, New York, Boston, Hartford, Lexington. It was in the large towns and cities that, first, mentally disordered persons needing attention became visible in too great a number for the informal methods of the village to deal with, and, second, there were enough enlightened people with the wealth and interest to attempt the provision of what was then considered therapeutic treatment in Europe, especially in England, which provided America with its models. As

Governor Francis Fauquier said in Williamsburg, all civilized nations had special hospitals for the mentally ill in which they could find asylum and proper medical care designed for their cure. This call for hospitals was less a condemnation of prevalent conditions (as was Dorothea Dix's crusade 75 years later) than a sign of growing faith in the ability of science to improve man's lot on earth.

In 1751, supporting Dr. Thomas Bond's appeal to Philadelphians to construct the first general hospital in the British North American colonies, the Pennsylvania Hospital, Benjamin Franklin discussed the need to include therein provision for the mentally ill. The incidence of insanity had not risen, he said, but the population had increased and with it the numbers of insane. Further, with the growth of Philadelphia into the leading city of the colonies, mental patients went there to be treated, presumably by physicians, but could not afford the high costs of lodging and nursing. It would appear that some rural people were searching for more effective care than was provided in the home and that they wanted something better than the available institutional alternatives. By this time those few laymen and physicians who were interested in mental disorder realized that jails, workhouses, and almshouses were undesirable repositories for persons whom they regarded as victims of some sort of disease of the brain and nervous system. Though many people came to regard general hospitals as places for the sick poor and the dying, this was much less the case with mental hospitals or the insane wards of general hospitals. In Philadelphia, for example, the Pennsylvania Hospital admitted mental patients from all social classes at the outset.

Almost a generation later, in 1766, Governor Fauquier urged the Virginia House of Burgesses to establish a mental hospital: "It is expedient I should . . . recommend to your Consideration and Humanity a poor unhappy set of People who are deprived of their Senses and wander about the country, terrifying the Rest of their Fellow Creatures. A legal Confinement, and proper Provision, ought to be appointed for these miserable Objects, who cannot help themselves. Every civilized Country has an Hospital for these People, where they are confined, maintained and attended by able Physicians, to endeavor to restore to them their lost Reason." *

* Virginia, General Assembly, House of Burgesses, *Journal*, Nov. 6, 1766, p. 12.

Fauquier died before his proposal, which the Burgesses approved, could be carried out, and his successor, Lord Botetourt, was moved to send four insane persons from Virginia prisons to the Pennsylvania Hospital at public expense. When the Burgesses finally founded the hospital in 1770, the preamble of the bill stated their reasons: "Whereas several persons of insane and disordered minds have been frequently found wandering in different parts of this colony, and no certain provision having been yet made either towards effecting a cure of those whose cases are not become quite desperate, nor for restraining others who may be dangerous to society. . . ." The governor, councilors, and Burgesses of the General Assembly then authorized the construction of a "public hospital, for the reception of such persons as shall, from time to time, according to the rules and orders established by this act, be sent thereto." * Actually, most of the patients received into the new hospital when it opened in 1773 and thereafter were not picked up from the streets and fields but were sent there by relatives who, if they could afford it, were supposed to pay for their keep.

Much the same attitudes were expressed in New York City by the organizers of the New York Hospital, the last of the three hospitals opened in the 18th century. One influential founder, Dr. Samuel Bard, knew of the work done among the insane at the Pennsylvania Hospital, probably through his physician father's friend, Benjamin Franklin, and also through contacts with the Philadelphia medical profession. He had studied in London, where, difficult as it may be to believe today, he was favorably impressed by what he saw at Bethlem (Bedlam) Hospital, and he wished to duplicate in New York the treatment given the insane there. Therefore, when New York Hospital opened in 1791, it had a psychiatric department.

These three small hospitals could accept only relatively few mental patients, and their operations were disrupted by the Revolution. Nevertheless, their establishment began in this country the custom of hospitalizing mentally disordered persons, a process greatly accelerated during the first half of the 19th century, widely adopted by the middle of the 20th, and then reversed by the 1960s. One may speculate that home care prevailed so

* William Waller Hening, ed., *The Statutes at Large; Being a Collection of All the Laws of Virginia from the First Session of the Legislature, in the Year 1619* (reprint ed., Charlottesville: University Press of Virginia, 1969), VIII: 378.

long not only because people resisted the surrender of friends and relatives to the care of strangers, but also because of the lack of alternative therapeutic or humane facilities. When such alternatives did become available, most of them, corporate or state establishments, quickly filled to capacity and then to overcapacity, albeit many people still distrusted hospitals and some communities found it cheaper—and keepers found it more profitable—to retain a patient in jail than to commit him to a mental hospital.

In a sense, even in the 18th century local communities were sequestering mental patients when they subsidized family care. A patient could be quite isolated at home, if only because the family was responsible for seeing that he or she caused no trouble; and keeping the patient inside the house and, if need be, under restraint, was the surest way to prevent unfortunate incidents. Further, mentally disordered people are disturbing to have around, perhaps less so on a farm or big plantation than in a cramped city dwelling, but still difficult to deal with, no matter how well family members cherish or understand them. Families would tend to want their patient out of sight or confined, not only because he could then do no harm to himself or others but also to spare themselves trouble. It is likely that most patients, then, did not have the freedom to be disruptive or to indulge their delusions fully. Family or home care did not necessarily signify any commitment to cure the insane or to integrate them into the community. Moreover, if, as has been hypothesized in our own day, family relationships can be crucial in the etiology of some mental disorders, how beneficial could even the best-intentioned home care have been? There are no grounds for romanticizing the lot of the insane given home care—much less the condition of those at large as vagabonds.

Whether hospital care was actually an improvement over home care is another question: to what extent did the early hospitals fulfill their therapeutic goals, and did they treat their patients well? Any such assessment should perhaps take into account current questions about mental illness being a true medical entity. If, as claimed, mental illness is altogether a social phenomenon, mental hospitals serve a function like that of prisons. They either reeducate deviants to conform, or, failing that, keep them out of circulation. If this view is accepted, mental hospitals never did perform traditional medical functions. Without entering into the substance of the argument—and without denying that it has been intellectually provocative and can be clinically fruitful in our contemporary psychiatric setting—one can say, first, that among those considered mentally ill in the past were persons suffering from what we know now as distinct pathological entities, the most significant one identified being syphilitic paresis. It is possible that other forms of mental disorders will be discovered to have chemical, genetic, or other somatic etiologies. Until we have conclusive evidence concerning the causes of most mental disorders it may be premature to exclude mental disease from traditional medical classification. Further, whatever the mix of social, psychological, and somatic factors may prove to be in mental disorders, it is evident that medicine has redefined the meaning of disease and continues to do so, so that the view of a fixed, enduring concept of illness to which mental disorder does not conform seems unwarranted.

In the 18th century, moreover, physicians and educated laymen, along with many others, considered insanity a somatic disorder not essentially different from any other—a disease of the brain and nervous system that in some unsatisfactorily explained way affected the mind, which was seen as quite separate from (though related to) the body. This viewpoint facilitated the replacement of the ancient moralistic-religious concepts of insanity by a clinical approach that offered the possibility of rational scientific treatment, in a revolution in psychiatry that even the best-known critic of contemporary psychiatry, R. D. Laing, has acknowledged. From a historical point of view, then, the early mental hospitals may be viewed and evaluated as medical institutions, although they performed "nonmedical" functions such as incarcerating dangerous or antisocial persons for the protection of society.

The physicians there did not have very much more to offer, however, than they had for patients suffering from other ailments. Following the prevalent English medical practice of heroic therapy, doctors bled, blistered, purged, drugged, and undernourished their mental patients; they bathed and showered them to reduce excitement, shocked and terrorized them to pull them out of stupor. At the Pennsylvania and New York hospitals, whips, chains, and camisoles were used to restrain agitated patients; in Williamsburg, patients were controlled by chains and straitjackets but were not whipped. Virtually no occupation or entertainment was offered, and in the Pennsylvania and New York hospitals housing conditions were very poor. Regarding insane patients as mere objects, physicians as well as laymen assumed that they did not feel extremes of cold or heat and that they were insensible to pain and other physical hardships. Moreover, while physicians made regular visits and prescribed and supervised treatment, day-to-day care was administered by lay keepers who varied in quality.

At the Pennsylvania Hospital, mental patients fared somewhat better after the famous Dr. Benjamin Rush took over the insane ward in 1789. He combined humane and rational care with his well-known reliance on bloodletting and other depletive measures. To replace traditional modes of restraint he invented a tranquilizing chair to keep the patient erect and immobile. Most of his practices were based on a mechanistic theory of pathology developed from ideas he had imbibed in Edinburgh and London. What he added—and what makes him a transitional figure in the history of psychiatry—was a concern for the mental state of the patient and a realization of the importance of kindness, decent accommodations, and the provision of some sort of occupation.

Practices at the New York Hospital resembled those at the Pennsylvania Hospital before Rush's ascendancy. Only in the 1820s, with the construction of its Bloomingdale Asylum and at the urging of Quaker businessman and philanthropist Thomas Eddy, were less heroic methods applied.

The Eastern State Hospital was somewhat different. Although traditional medical remedies were inflicted upon patients by the attending physicians, life seems to have been more pleasant there, perhaps because of the warmer climate and bucolic setting, and because the hospital was small and run by a prominent local family, the Galts, who had a reputation for kindness. Two branches of the family devoted themselves to the patients for almost 100 years, one branch supplying lay keepers, the other, physicians and medical superintendents. Further, although Williamsburg was the capital of Virginia until 1780, it was always a small place in which the hospital was a major industry, and since everyone knew everyone else, any cruelty and mistreatment of patients would become common knowledge. The Eastern State Hospital was unique in being entirely under government sponsorship (the only hospital so sponsored in the United States for almost 50 years) and open to all, regardless of color, class, or ability to pay (with the apparent exception of slaves until the 1840s). The other early asylums were voluntary institutions established through state charters, and, although usually in receipt of public funds, they were not freely open to the public.

All the early hospitals not only hoped to return patients to the community as restored or improved, but did so, although such success is difficult to evaluate. The interpretation of "cured" or "restored" is variable, the types of patients and their symptoms have changed, and many factors other than treatment in the hospital are involved in the reported outcome of therapy. However, one rough, highly simplified criterion can perhaps be used. It is my contention that, for the past several centuries, therapeutically oriented mental hospitals with conditions at least minimally decent by contemporary standards, in England, France, the United States, Canada, and probably also in Spain and Italy, have returned approximately one-third of their patients to the community as cured. These appear to have been "spontaneous" recoveries. Another third remained chronically ill, and the last third improved in varying degrees, many to the point of being discharged. The not infrequent reports by 18th-century hospitals of recoveries of between 20 to 30 percent indicate that they were more than simply custodial institutions, and that there must have been some commitment to curing patients.

Still, 18th-century psychiatry had really nowhere to go if physicians continued to prescribe the conventional remedies that scarcely worked for any other illness, much less for insanity. With all their best efforts it was unlikely that more than the already claimed one-quarter to one-third of their patients could be "restored" under the prevailing somatic regimens; they could do little more than create conditions that permitted such "spontaneous" recoveries. Yet because of their exclusively somatic training and the struggle the medical profession had had to place mental illness under its aegis, to convince the public to take a clinical rather than a supernatural view, most physicians remained wedded to a narrow somatic therapeutic system that yielded few results then and for generations thereafter. The symptoms might be mental or emotional, but the underlying pathology had to be physical and so the therapy was physical. Otherwise, not only might the insane have to be yielded up again to exorcists, but the possibility that the immortal soul might be diseased would have to be considered, in a challenge to conventional Christian theology that most physicians preferred not to issue. So, in keeping to a strict mind-body dichotomy, they were, as they saw it, protecting the medical profession, their mental patients, and hallowed religious concepts all at the same time.

The conversion of the enlightened humanitarian impulse of the 18th century into a new humanistic therapeutic system came from devout Quaker laymen in England, and radical physicians like Pinel in revolutionary France, who were, for different reasons, unperturbed by the implications of medicine and science for theology. They represented in their thinking two unorthodox philosophical strains that saved them from the ambivalence felt by conventional medical men and freed them to take a fresh approach: the Quaker's emotional, individualistic religious belief that regarded all men as equal and all souls as saved, and Pinel's skeptical rationalism that considered religion irrelevant to medicine. Both views were humanistic though disparate, and both groups were very practical. Working separately, they arrived at similar results—the regimen that became known as moral treatment, to which Rush also made independent contributions. It was an approach that made the optimism itself the therapy, that transferred the concern for the mentally ill as a class into a concern for them as individuals. Although the traditional medical therapies were not wholly discarded, the emphasis was on kindness, compassion, consideration, warmth, good company, freedom of movement, occupation, recreation, the elimination of physical punishment, appeals to the moral sense, persuasion, and training in good habits and self-control. Hospitals were to be in a rural setting with considerable acreage not so much to isolate patients as to afford them healthful living, space in which to roam, land on which they could busy themselves gardening or farming, and freedom from disturbing relatives and prying neighbors. Such provision was seen as a vital aspect of treatment, indispensable to the cure as well as the comfort of patients. It was not merely that common humanity dictated benevolence, as in the hospital at Williamsburg, but that benevolence was a prerequisite for recovery.

In the United States, although Rush's influence was very real, the major force in the introduction of moral treatment was the work of a Quaker family, the Tukes, who established in the 1790s the famous York Retreat in England, upon which several new American corporate institutions were modeled: the Friends' Asylum (now the Friends' Hospital) outside Philadelphia, opened in 1817; McLean Asylum near Boston, opened in 1819; and the Hartford Retreat (now the Institute of Living), opened in 1824. In the 1820s one of the older hospitals, the New York Hospital, initiated moral treatment under Quaker influence, and several state hospitals built in the 1830s and 1840s instituted it. At the Pennsylvania and Eastern State hospitals the change was not fully made until the early 1840s.

The moral treatment movement, which claimed recoveries up to 60 percent and more, lasted until about the time of the Civil War, when it gradually lapsed into oblivion, only to be designated by recent historians as a progressive aspect of what had been considered an unrelievedly bleak past. It was a time when belief in curability was high; patients fortunate enough to be admitted to the best hospitals, named asylums or retreats according to their philosophy, could live in an environment that was humane, decent, and designed to make them feel better. The new system was such a marked improvement that it cast its 18th-century antecedents into the shade. Yet, although moral treatment was a break with the past it was at the same time a logical outcome of it, originating as it did in the optimism of the Enlightenment and in the ideal of clinical treatment of the mentally ill that stimulated the creation of the first mental hospitals, with one of them, the Eastern State Hospital, a pioneer in its state sponsorship and open admissions policy. Further, men like Benjamin Rush, for all his passion for phlebotomy, did extend the concept of therapy beyond the narrow somaticism of the past. The greatest distinction, then, between the two periods was that the early 19th century saw the implementation of concepts that had arisen in the 18th.

Superseding these eras of reform was a long spell, from the mid-19th to the mid-20th century, during which therapeutic pessimism, custodialism, and bureaucracy prevailed in most mental hospitals. The de-humanizing conditions there were described and condemned in classic accounts by reformers like Clifford Beers in 1908 and Albert Deutsch in the 1940s; reformers and radicals in our own day have been struggling to change them. The introduction of milieu therapy or the therapeutic environment in the

1950s, followed by the community mental health movement, was in some ways a return to the moral treatment of over a century earlier.

The history of the treatment of mental illness, then, is not that of a benighted past evolving into the enlightened present. Although a cumulative element cannot be denied, the historical pattern tends to be more cyclic than linear. Mental hospitals have exhibited fluctuations in their practices, at times being the most tolerable and in some cases the most desirable refuges for the mentally disordered, at other times, highly intolerable and undesirable. The evidence does not support a claim that all of necessity are — and always have been — essentially custodial, a means of social control; nor does it substantiate the belief that state mental hospitals were always gigantic machines for sequestering aberrant individuals and rendering them harmless. It is inappropriate, therefore, to read back into history the problems of a later day. To deny the positive contributions of early hospitals and the humanistic motives of their founders and managers in order to justify the censure of modern institutions may be understandable politics, but it is poor history.

Bibliography

Altschule, M. D.: *Roots of Modern Psychiatry: Essays in the History of Psychiatry.* 2d (rev. and enlarged) ed. New York: Grune & Stratton, 1905.

Blackmon, D. M. E.: *The Care of the Mentally Ill in America, 1604–1812, in the Thirteen Original Colonies.* Ph.D. dissertation, University of Washington, 1964.

Braceland, F. J.: *The Institute of Living, The Hartford Retreat, 1822–1972.* Hartford, Conn.: The Institute of Living, 1972.

Dain, N.: *Concepts of Insanity in the United States, 1789–1865.* New Brunswick, N.J.: Rutgers University Press, 1964.

——: *Disordered Minds: The First Century of Eastern State Hospital in Williamsburg, Virginia, 1766–1866.* Williamsburg, Va.: The Colonial Williamsburg Foundation, 1971.

Deutsch, A.: *The Mentally Ill in America: A History of Their Care and Treatment from Colonial Times.* Garden City, N.Y.: Doubleday, Doran, 1937.

Eaton, L. K.: *New England Hospitals, 1790–1833.* Ann Arbor: University of Michigan Press, 1957.

Grob, G. N.: *The State and the Mentally Ill: A History of Worcester State Hospital in Massachusetts, 1830–1920.* Chapel Hill: University of North Carolina Press, 1966.

——: *Mental Institutions in America: Social Policy to 1875.* New York: Free Press, 1973.

Hurd, H. N. (ed.) : *The Institutional Care of the Insane in the United States and Canada.* (4 vols.) Baltimore: The Johns Hopkins Press, 1916–17.

Laing, R. D., and Esterson, A.: *Sanity, Madness, and the Family.* Harmondsworth, England: Penguin Books, 1964, p. 27.

Leigh, D.: *The Historical Development of British Psychiatry.* Vol. 1: *18th and 19th Century.* New York: Pergamon Press, 1961.

Morton, T. G.: *The History of the Pennsylvania Hospital, 1751–1895.* Rev. ed. Philadelphia: Times Printing House, 1897.

One Hundred Years of American Psychiatry. New York: Columbia University Press, for the American Psychiatric Association, 1944.

Pinel, P.: *A Treatise on Insanity.* Trans. D. D. Davis. New York: Hafner Publishing Company, under the auspices of the Library of the New York Academy of Medicine, 1962. A facsimile of the London 1806 edition.

Rosen, G.: *Madness in Society: Chapters in the Historical Sociology of Mental Illness.* Chicago: University of Chicago Press, 1968.

Rothman, D. J.: *The Discovery of the Asylum: Social Order and Disorder in the New Republic.* Boston: Little, Brown, 1971.

Rush, B.: *Medical Inquiries and Observations upon the Diseases of the Mind.* Philadelphia: Kimber & Richardson, 1812.

Russell, W. L.: *The New York Hospital: A History of the Psychiatric Service, 1771–1936.* New York: Columbia University Press, 1945.

Tuke, S.: *Description of the Retreat, an Institution Near York for the Insane Persons of the Society of Friends. . . .* York: Printed for W. Alexander, London, 1813.

5. *American Psychiatry: Past, Present, and Future*

Keynote Address

John Romano, M.D.

IT IS said that each generation is apt to overestimate its contribution to its time. Regrettably, we cannot know what were the hopes or the claims of John deSequeyra, who cared for the mad 200 years ago, and who, among others, we honor today in this bicentenary celebration. Naturally we wonder what he thought of what we consider today to be the harsh, restrictive physical measures and the heroic pharmacology of his time—jalap and calomel, opium and camphor, sassafras and antimony.

We are more fortunate, thanks to the scholarship of Professor Dain (1971), in our knowledge of the work of John Minson Galt II, who assumed responsibility for the superintendency of the Eastern Lunatic Asylum almost 50 years after deSequeyra's death. Although Galt continued to use the traditional medical measures of his day, narcotics and tonics and purgatives, with occasional bloodletting, he also introduced measures associated with moral treatment. These included the substitution of kindness for harsh measures, and the amelioration of isolation through the creation of social situations like those enjoyed by the healthy and sane. This attitude toward the mad had been revived at the end of the 18th century by Chiarugi, Pinel, and Tuke from ancient Greek and Roman writings. As we look back and read about jalap and sassafras, whether with sympathy and understanding or with a gentle patronizing smile, should we not ask ourselves how those who follow after us will look on our efforts? If our cumulative libraries of books, journals, and pamphlets, audio- and videotapes, and movie films are not disastrously lost, our successors should have little trouble in learning about our activities and the beliefs, judgments, and notions that underlie our practices. They may indeed find an embarrassment of riches. We may think of ourselves as long-suffering, but I feel others look upon us as long-winded; and when we listen carefully to ourselves we must be reminded of Elting Morison's remark, "The smaller the understanding of the situation, the more pretentious, often, the form of expression."

Will our successors understand and respect what we have tried to do? As far as I know, neither jalap or sassafras is used extensively at the moment, certainly not in the treatment of the mentally sick, but will our successors smile indulgently or frown with perplexity when they read of seemingly infinite psychoanalytic treatment addictions; of the crotch eyeballing in group therapies; of the megavitamins; of the retribalization of family network therapy; of concern with the games people play and when one person stamps another as OK; of certain aspects of psychosurgery; of the indiscriminate use of medication; of bumbling political intervention in ventures for community mental health? We will never know what they will think, but we can use this moment to examine as best we can what we believe to be our achievements, and where we think they may take us in the next several years.

Would we not all agree at the outset that we have *not* achieved an understanding of the basic causes and mechanisms of mental illness? Nevertheless, American psychiatry has changed since World War II, largely because of the passage in 1946 of the National Mental Health Law sponsored by the 79th Congress. This made possible generous financial support for related education and research. In my view the past 25 years will be looked upon by tomorrow's historians as being a significant and critical period in the history of our profession. I say this knowing that from our early beginnings there have been other periods during which great expectations of our knowledge and skills were entertained. I have already referred to the period of moral treatment, which was in accord with the Humanitarian Movement of the late 19th century, and which, in the United States, was followed by the cult of curability and the establishment of state institutions.

The mental hygiene movement, born in the first decade of this century, reflected much of our characteristic American evangelical optimism and pragmatism. It was followed by the child guidance movement after World War I. This was to be the century of the child! At about the same time a number of psychiatric observation wards and psychopathic hospitals were established, usually intimately associated with university medical centers. Early in the century they were built in Albany, Ann

Arbor, Boston, and Baltimore, and, later on, in Denver, Iowa City, and New York. Each was intended to receive all types of mentally ill persons for observation and examination, and to provide short intensive treatment of acutely ill patients. From these centers outpatient treatment was begun, albeit initially on a modest scale. These institutions, together with a few large private hospitals and several even larger state mental hospitals, were the principal theaters for the beginnings of the systematic education of career psychiatrists and laboratory and investigative clinical work.

Still another movement was that of psychoanalysis and the emergence of the social sciences, to which America gave warm welcome although the giants, the creative innovators in these fields, were, for the most part, European.

There are likely to be differences among us as to what we consider the most important contributions of our time, but may I indicate those I consider most significant? These are not necessarily listed in order of importance, and in several instances I am speaking of trends rather than of something actually already achieved: (1) the establishment of psychiatric units in general teaching and community hospitals; (2) the teaching of psychiatry to all undergraduate medical students; (3) the considerable enlargement of the manpower pool of career psychiatrists through resident teaching programs, in university and affiliated clinics and hospitals, that provide psychiatrists for private and group community practices; (4) the furtherance of research through educational opportunities in research at NIMH and the university departments of psychiatry; (5) the introduction of psychology and the social sciences into the matrix of the medical school teaching hospital; (6) multiple ventures in psychotherapeutic procedures, from psychoanalytic origins to diverse group and family techniques, from learning theory to behavior modification, and to several combinations of these; (7) the extensive use of the major psychoactive drugs in the treatment of psychotic patients, and the use of minor tranquilizers by the general practitioner in the treatment of neurotic conditions; (8) the growth of the general practice of psychiatry as well as the more restrictive therapeutic special practices, and the role of such general practices in returning the care of the chronically ill patient from the state to the local community; (9) the expansion of educational programs for psychiatric nurses and psychiatric social workers, and their assumption of new roles in therapy and care; (10) the creation of new types of paraprofessional persons in child and adult care—nursing assistants, mental health workers, etc., who participate at many points in the health service network; (11) the beginning of systematic studies into the nature of health delivery systems—emergency care, triage determinations, neighborhood centers, home visiting, outpatient and inpatient clinics, and chronic hospitals, and the remarkable changes in patient distribution from inpatient to outpatient services, etc.; (12) attention to areas of neglect—the chronically sick, the poor, the black, the addict, the alcoholic, and the criminal; (13) expansion of child psychiatry beyond its traditional engagement with the middle class neurotic child into wider concerns for children with brain damage, psychosis, retardation, and delinquent behavior; (14) increased interest in and attention to human genetics, to biological studies of mind and brain, and mind and body; (15) greater precision in clinical diagnosis in the course of illness, with greater attention to the physical examination of the patient.

Perhaps because of my sustained major interest in education, and because the future of the profession depends on how its young are prepared, I believe that one of the most important contributions psychiatry has made to medicine since World War II is the education of the medical student—that is, of all physicians whether or not their major concern in later life is in patient care. On previous occasions I have noted (Romano 1973) that it has become possible for the medical student today to study and care for mentally sick patients in the same hospital setting in which he studied medical, surgical, and obstetrical patients. This has been made possible during the past 25 years largely by federal subsidies, through the establishment of psychiatric units in general teaching hospitals and the appointment of full-time or part-time clinical psychiatric faculties in medical schools. In 1972 there were 2,500 full-time psychiatric faculty appointments. Thirty years ago there were fewer than 200.

It is in the general hospital that the student has learned to identify, to understand, to be responsible for, and to treat a broad range of distressed patients who may be delirious or demented, depressed or hypochondriacal, and to learn something of the great enigma that is schizophrenia. This is quite unlike my experience, more than 40 years ago, which was made up of two visits to a chronic hospital, and a sonorously dull lecture series. It is in the general hospital that the student becomes aware of the universality of suicidal ideas, the frequency of suicide attempts, and the fact that suicide is a major cause of death. In this setting he also learns something of current theories and practices of care and treatment, medication, psychotherapy, and family therapy as they relate to emergency, crisis, short-term, and long-term hospital care; and it is here, too, that he rediscovers the fact that man is a social animal, that his patient is a member of a group, of a family, and that the patient's distress and symptoms can be understood more clearly if they are dealt with in these social terms.

Similarly, the student learns that he, too, is a member of a group in the hospital, and in this way he learns more specifically of his role, the tasks assigned to him, and those assigned to his associates. The student's assignments in the traditional teaching hospital give him an unusual opportunity to learn of the psychology of illness and disability, and the coping capacities of patients with handicaps. He learns something of the psychology of pain, of fatigue, of ennui and depression, and he can learn of the events, including bereavement, that take place in those who care for the dying patient. Skill in objective observation has been his principal heritage from his background in physical and biological science, but he can learn other types of observation, namely those of participant observation, subjective observation, and self-observation, and in doing this he learns something of his role in the human encounter between the patient and himself and between members of the patient's family, and he learns that this differentiation of his role is necessary for a better understanding of his relationship to his patient and his growing capacity for human intimacy in the specific task of becoming a physician. Perhaps for the first time the student is confronted with the fact that there is no satisfactory unitary concept of human biology, and that, in spite of the valiant attempts of general systems theorists, there has emerged no satisfactory language to do full justice to the biological, psychological, and social aspects of the human condition. He does learn the general notion of personality and the basic principles that underlie understanding: genic and ontogenetic factors in growth, development, and decline; the recognition of unconscious and preconscious factors as determinants of behavior; the idea that the personality is integral and indivisible; and the psychosocial principle that recognizes that man is a social animal and that the emerging stages of the life cycle must be understood in terms of the crucial coordination between the developing individual and his social environment. I believe all this has led to a clearer concept of health and disease and to the regretful realization that psychopathology survives and prospers under many flags. The fallacy of the single cause is nowhere more obvious than in considerations of health and disease. These, then, are among the advantages today's students have over their predecessors. Obviously, many bodies of knowledge, including psychoanalytic psychology, have played their parts in helping today's physician obtain a better understanding of the patient and his family. Since I see such training as a substantial contribution to the physician's education, it is small wonder that I am seriously concerned about the current trend to reduce the undergraduate period by a year, to establish multiple tracks of curriculum early in the student's experience, and to diminish opportunities for broad general clinical scholarship.

What of the psychiatrist's education? As in medicine before World War II, in psychiatry there were few residency programs and few residents in each. The system was quite informal and fundamentally based on the preceptorship model used for interns and residents in medicine at Johns Hopkins at the beginning of the century. With the exponential increase in the number of programs—80 in 1927 and 400 in 1972—and the number of residents—400 in 1927 and 5,859 in 1972—much of the informal intimacy of the educational program has been lost.* Forty years ago (in 1933) the American Psychiatric Association had 1,517 members; in 1945, at the end of World War II, it had 3,634. In the last count available, that of 1971, the total membership was 19,037. I believe there are more psychiatrists today than there are pediatricians or obstetricians. John Cotton of St. Luke's Hospital in New York told me recently that there are more practicing psychiatrists in New York City than there are general practitioners

---

* Since the reading of this paper Dr. Walter Barton updated these figures and indicated that as of September 1, 1972, there were 4,750 residents in training. Ninety percent were in the first three years of training, and 10 percent were in advanced training, most in child psychiatry. There were 288 approved residency programs and 15 other programs presently inactive or being deactivated. Nine of these were in state mental hospitals or in the Veterans Administration.

of medicine. Forty years ago, even in large cities, most, if not all, psychiatrists served on the staffs of mental hospitals, the majority being attached to public institutions. There may have been a small number at work in child guidance clinics, the growth of which came after World War I; and an even smaller number engaged in forensic work in local civil and criminal courts. Few were involved in the private practice of psychiatry in the community as separate from a position on a hospital staff. It was the general practitioner, the internist, and the neurologist who saw and cared for the many patients, principally neurotic persons, who are now cared for by the psychiatrist. Teaching programs were to be found before World War II in several state hospitals, university-based psychopathic hospitals with limited outpatient service, and a few distinguished private mental hospitals.

For purposes of comparison my experiences (Romano 1970a) in a university-based psychopathic hospital almost 40 years ago may be of interest. After a year's general internship and a first year in clinical psychiatry at Yale with Eugen Kahn, I served as Resident Commonwealth Fellow at the University of Colorado from 1935 to 1938. The major thrust of the program was our daily engagement in the study, care, and treatment of patients who suffered from a broad spectrum of psychopathological conditions, but we were, in addition, exposed to and involved in occasionally dramatic medical-legal issues, consultative services to courts and social agencies, demonstration child-and-adult clinics in nearby small towns, and diagnostic and treatment services to a nearby institution for delinquent boys, with three- to four-month assignments to the state hospital 100 miles distant, and many educational lectures to parent-teacher and lay organizations in our city and throughout the state. We had just begun to take part in liaison activity between psychiatry and the medical, surgical, and obstetrical services in the university's general hospital.

We were involved in the therapies enthusiastically proposed at that time, with dauerschlaf (prolonged narcosis) and insulin, with pentavalent arsenicals and the Kettering hypertherm used to treat patients with neurosyphilis. We used chloral and bromides and the barbiturates as wisely as we knew how, and we practiced the various types of insight and supportive psychotherapies then available. Sulpha had arrived but penicillin was yet to come, and we would wait another 20 years before chlorpromazine became available. Later in our stay, metrazol was used, and ECT was on the horizon. We seemed to have an endless number of acutely disturbed patients, and along with the nurses and attendants we responded to their emergency needs with the gusto of seasoned firehorses.

There was little or no formal instruction as we know it today in the form of tutorials, seminars, conferences, and sequential lectures. We taught and learned from one another and at times had long and heated discussions about the diagnosis and understanding of our patients, and the appropriate treatment for them. I do remember our pervasive concern for the history of ideas and the origins of our then current theories and practices. We used the library frequently and intensively and started our own journal club. The neural sciences were poorly taught, but we did see neurologic patients. Later I obtained more systematic training at Harvard as a Rockefeller Fellow in Neurology. Psychology and social work were represented by a few valiant souls who served principally as handmaidens, in a situation remote from the rich and profitable interchange that engages psychology, social work, and psychiatry today in most university departments. Several of us were seriously interested in teaching; we vied with one another for assignments to teach medical students.

We grew up using the outline for psychiatric examination that was prepared by Clarence Cheney, derived from George Kirby and, before Kirby, from Adolf Meyer. In Colorado, John Benjamin, freshly arrived from Zurich and from his association with the Bleulers and Emile Oberholzer, shared with us his interest in and knowledge of psychoanalysis and the Rorschach. He spoke to us of cognitive disturbances and other thought disorders of schizophrenic patients and of the general temper of Continental psychiatry. As I remember it, little formal investigative work was carried on, although several of us did become involved in clinical case histories and follow-up studies. There were, in fact, no models of scientific investigators available to us. At that time psychiatry had no Rockefeller Institute to help groom its young professors, as was the case in medicine and physiology. We had to wait almost 15 years before NIMH became a reality. Our models were the clinician-teacher-scholar and, later the psychoanalytic-psychotherapist-practitioner. Today we have additional models, including the clinician-investigator and a new mutation, the behavioral scientist. We realized that our knowledge and our various practices stemmed from belief systems and bodies of knowledge that did not permit any unified concept. I am not sure that this troubled us too much, as our primary loyalty was to our patients and there seemed to be so much to learn. Through our study of the patients entrusted to us, our study among ourselves, and our reading, we were exposed to those notions, concepts, and bodies of knowledge thought to be relevant to the acquisition of the clinical psychiatrist's skills—human genetics, the neural sciences, human growth and development, psychodynamics and psychopathology, clinical psychology (principally psychometrics), a smattering of sociology, the clinical syndromes, diagnosis, course, prognosis, epidemiology, and the limited therapeutic approaches of the day. We read and studied from several American and English textbooks as well as translations of E. Bleuler and E. Kraepelin. We read the journals and were aware that Kraepelin, Freud, Adolf Meyer, Harry Stack Sullivan, Kempf, Karl Menninger, William Alanson White, and several others had contributed to our education.

Although the basic system of most resident programs has remained pluralistic, there were and are many variations, with some programs emphasizing the biologic and pharmacologic aspects of the field, and others, the psychologic or social. In this century, psychiatry has been influenced by Kraepelin's descriptive school of clinical psychiatry, including the genetic and biochemical implications; by the contributions of social psychologists and sociologists, particularly Talcott Parsons; by the contributions of psychoanalytic psychology and various derivative psychotherapeutic techniques, especially the uniquely American ventures into group and family therapies; and by learning theory. From these several sources, as Redlich and Freedman (1966) have pointed out, two theories became influential, one being the motivational theory that emerged from Freud's study of neurotic patients. This notion draws attention to the conflict of competing needs and drives for expression, or compromise solutions of these needs. The second, more familiar to medicine, is the traditional neurobiological theory that stresses deficits, impaired capacities, release or loss of controlled behavior, and the lowering of the organizational level.

Each has had its past. In the mists of antiquity one can find allegations that disease or sickness may be related to fear, to shame, or to guilt, or to feelings of having done wrong; on the other hand, we can trace our neurobiological concept of brain pathology back at least to Hippocrates. It seems obvious that both concepts are necessary to the intelligent study of the etiology of any behavior disorder, but I have on other occasions drawn attention to the uniquely significant impact of psychoanalysis on American (as contrasted with European) psychiatry, which led to a polarization of belief systems among us. That is, some retain a genetic, biological model of behavior, but others champion a psychosocial model. This development led to the engagement of a considerable number of psychiatrists, as well as psychoanalysts, in private psychotherapeutic practices based on psychoanalytic principles and concerned principally with neurotic middle class patients. Furthermore, the nature of the neurotic distress treated has changed from that of symptom distress—that is, symptom neurosis—to that of character neurosis. Although many psychoanalysts have taken part in the education of medical students and psychiatric residents, particularly in the supervision of such students in psychotherapeutic ventures, many have remained quite distant from the study and care of the psychotic patient, as well as from the mainstream of general medicine.

Psychiatrists in the psychiatric units of general teaching hospitals became available for consultative purposes on the other clinical floors of their hospitals. Several liaison programs between psychiatry and medicine and psychiatry and pediatrics were developed, and serious attempts were made to search for specificity in the emotional life-style of patients with somatic illnesses, often called psychosomatic. The attempts were not notably successful in determining specificity, although many of the studies assisted the physician to understand and manage his patients better. The psychiatric units of general hospitals made possible the study and care of the occasional neurotic patient who required hospital admission, but the principal service function of the psychiatric unit has been the study and care of the acutely psychotic patient or the chronic patient in an exacerbation of his illness. Thus one saw many depressed persons and many schizophrenic patients. A broad range of diagnostic and therapeutic procedures was used, including individual and group psychotherapy, family therapy, milieu treatment, behavior modification, physical treatment like ECT, and, since 1954, psychotropic drugs. Systematic clinical research was supported generously by federal funds, but few in psychiatry have been hospitable to or greatly interested in the alcoholic, the addict, the aged, and the chronically mentally sick.

Thus today's psychiatrists are unlike those of 40 years ago, when the few psychiatrists there were served almost exclusively in public or private mental hospitals. Today's psychiatrists work principally in community, private, or group practices; in clinics and general hospitals, including those for children and adolescents; in schools, courts, and agencies; on the faculties of our medical schools; and at the National Institute of Mental Health.

Nevertheless, one senses change in the air. I predict that in this last third of the century we shall be increasingly concerned with psychosis, in a change from that greater concern with neurosis which, as I haved noted, occupied the attention of most of us in the middle third of the century. The reasons for my belief are several. Our current mood or ambience of concern about civil rights, privacy, and commitment draws attention to areas of human neglect, including the care provided the psychotic patient. This focus is implicit in the development of community mental health programs with the deliberate and conscious recognition that we must acquire systematic knowledge of the delivery of health services. It is the moral treatment of our day. The community programs have led to the increasing visibility of the psychotic and society's greater tolerance of him in the community. The effectiveness of ECT and, in the past 15 years, of psychotropic drugs has enabled many of us to reduce the distress of psychotic patients and in many instances to enhance their social competence. There has been a renaissance of biochemistry, pharmacology, and genetics as these relate to the field of psychiatry, and, with this, the recruitment and support of top-drawer researchers in these fields. There is greater concern for precision in diagnosis as it has become necessary now to discriminate carefully among schizophrenia, mania, the several types of depression, and other psychotic behavior in order to prescribe the appropriate medication. The emphasis in research into depressive disorders has shifted away from consideration of psychologic phenomena toward the biological aspects of the disease. In the study of schizophrenia, research continues to probe psychosocial as well as biological parameters. The daily use of medication has required continuing physical—as well as psychologic—screening of patients, and the psychiatrist has had to become familiar with certain laboratory methods in order to gauge drug dosage and to avoid toxic complications. Psychiatrists are being advised by pharmacologists and clinicians as to appropriate prescribing patterns and the need to individualize medication treatment and to avoid polypharmacy.

There are those who believe that this trend constitutes a neo-Kraepelinian movement characterized by consideration of genetic factors as significant determinants of illness, by greater precision in noting signs and symptoms of disease, by the charting of the natural course of illness, and by follow-up studies of the effects of intervention on prognosis. It draws attention to the neurobiological model as well as to the motivational model as a determinant of illness. In short, the psychiatrist is returning to being a doctor.

There are other trends. There has emerged a more sober view of the efficacy of analytic psychotherapy, disenchantment with its earlier claims of success, and, perhaps most important, the feeling that it seems to be stuck on a conceptual basis with very few germinal ideas emerging. As in economics, there has been no fresh theoretical idea of consequence for over 40 years. As Katz (1970) has pointed out, psychotherapy appears to have branched out from a setting of pervasive psychodynamic psychoanalytic notions into two movements quite opposite from one another. One is that of behavior modification, derived from Pavlov, Hull, and Skinner. In this there are highly rational goal-directed procedures that emphasize the shaping and control of behavior through cognitive methods or through laboratory principles of learning. These techniques can be defined with precision, as can the criteria of success. Central in behavior modification is the notion of control. The therapist clearly states the nature and direction of the procedure.

Quite opposite to behavior modification is a whole set of group techniques which includes the encounter method, the sensitivity techniques, and Gestalt therapy. These appear to represent affective or feeling tone. The general orientation is toward release of inner controls and the liberation of feelings and of previously suppressed aspects of the personality. As in psychoanalytic therapy, the processes through which these techniques work are not clearly definable, nor are the therapists very precise about the goals to be achieved. The critical element seems to be to expand the awareness of the individual to help him acknowledge dissociated aspects of his personality, and to reunite the mind and body within the overall therapeutic experience. In therapeutic practice much of what has developed in each of these opposing movements has come from psychologists as well as psychiatrists. These group techniques are often used in crash training programs for those new types of professional or paraprofessional persons who would be prepared more briefly to do, perhaps at lower cost, some of the things the psychiatrist has been doing. We find counselors for drug abusers, alcoholics, and migrant workers taking their part in community mental health programs, providing continuing care of patients and a broad spectrum of services considered appropriate to the patients' needs. I draw your attention to this development because I believe that many persons other than psychiatrists—psychologists, social workers, and paraprofessional mental health workers, for example—will be increasingly involved in individual and group psychotherapeutic procedures in the future. I believe, too, that the general physician, including the internist, will continue to be active in the identification and treatment of most neurotic patients in his practice because of his undergraduate educational experience in psychiatry, and that he will be aided in his practice by the judicious use of the minor tranquilizers, librium and valium.

As you well know, there is yet another trend, that of the community mental health program. In a sense, this is a vanguard movement of something that will be taking place in all of medicine. It reflects our increasing concern with the delivery of health services, with the awareness of our current deficiencies in the continuity of patient care, and with the search for measures that may best serve our patients' needs. It has led some to insist that the major objective of psychiatry in education, research, and service should be that of primary prevention—that is, the psychiatrist should become informed about and socially and politically active in reducing poverty, overpopulation, and racial discrimination, and in improving education, employment, and housing. Obviously, this would be a major departure from our traditional educational patterns, which are based on our concern for and care of the individual. It would imply an objective more oriented to public health. There seems little question that we are to be more concerned with chronic illness in all of medicine. Our traditional model, at least from the beginning of this century, has been the identification, treatment, and prevention of acute infectious disease, and I believe this was an appropriate model for the first third or perhaps the first half of the century; but today the major problems of almost all of medicine are those of chronic illness. Certainly it is the major problem in psychiatry. I recently learned that in the Veterans Administration system alone there are 5,000 schizophrenic men who have been hospitalized 10 years or more. This point was made vivid to me when, on February 6, 1973, a party was held for 22 men patients in the Canandaigua Veterans Administration Hospital, with which I have been associated. These 22 patients had come with 200 others when the hospital was opened 40 years ago, on February 6, 1933. Twenty of the 22 have retained the diagnosis of schizophrenia.

And so we see these trends moving toward clinical medicine and biologic research; toward new ventures in psychotherapy and the increasing of the pool of professional and paraprofessional persons to be engaged in psychotherapy; toward involvement with social public health and health service delivery, with increasing concern for the chronically ill, for prevention—and the ever-present search for understanding of the basic causes and mechanisms of mental illness underlying all the rest. Would it not seem sensible, then, to attempt to educate tomorrow's physicians and psychiatrists in such a way that they may be optimally prepared to meet the issues and challenges of their day? There are trends in the educational programs for residents, as well as in those offered medical students, that would limit the future psychiatrist's contribution to his own field as well as to other areas of medical practice. The elimination of the free-standing internship and the truncation of the period of residency comes at a time of imperative need to deal with a considerable increase of knowledge concerning biologic, psychologic, and social aspects of human behavior, and at a time when our federal government has decided to reduce materially its support of the educational program (Romano 1970b).

Thoughtful colleagues have commented that confusion about their identity has been recognized by psychiatrists as a problem at least since World War II (Brody 1972). Similar confusion may be evident in the psychiatric profession in other nations (Meijering and Dekker 1973). It seems unlikely that whatever confusion there may be could result from the fact that there is, as yet, no satisfactory unitary concept which encompasses human behavior in biological, psychological, and social terms; certainly this dilemma has been with us for a long time, and I would expect it to be with us for some time to come. Is not whatever confusion there is more likely a reflection of the very considerable changes taking place in our nation in the whole matrix of medical, educational, research, and clinical services in all disciplines? More particularly, is not our confusion related to the fact that there are now many persons, paraprofessional as well as professional—psychologists, social workers, social scientists, nurses, mental health counselors, etc.—who are assuming duties formerly discharged exclusively by psychiatrists?

In addition to whatever professional identity confusion there may be, there is also criticism and question from within the profession and from outside. There are those who believe that psychiatry has not responded to the needs of the poor, the black, the chronic psychotic, the addict, the criminal, and the subnormal, including the brain-damaged child. It is said that the modern physician, particularly the psychotherapist-psychiatrist, is apt to choose as his patients those whom he most resembles, and as many of us are middle class, white, and verbal, so are the patients we see. Voltaire said, "If a camel had a God, it would probably look something like a camel." What is evident is that besides the criticism that arises from within and without are what are called antipsychiatry movements. It appears to me that a profession can only benefit from criticism; in the past we benefited materially from the trenchant critiques of Weir Mitchell, Alan Gregg, Roy Grinker, Percival Bailey, and others. You will remember that Shaw remarked that every profession is a conspiracy against society. In the long run, society determines the professions it chooses to serve it.

Is it not our responsibility to examine our role, our function, what it is that we do? I believe that the major function of psychiatry, and one unique to it, is to serve as a crucial bridge connecting genetics, biology, and clinical medicine on the one hand, and the behavioral sciences on the other. The psychologist, the social worker, and the social scientist lack knowledge of the body; the biologist lacks knowledge of the mind; and, up to the present, the nurse has had insufficient education in either field to bridge them. Further, I believe that if we are to serve this function properly, we must not only reaffirm our fundamental membership in medicine but we must become informed with the contributions of our colleagues in the behavioral sciences. To neglect scholarship at either pole would be to diminish our usefulness for tomorrow. We cannot afford to neglect the promising and interesting developments occurring in genetics, in biochemistry and physiology, and pharmacology, all of which are relevant to our task; nor can we afford to overlook what psychologists, social scientists, and economists can offer to help us understand the full dimensions of man in human and social terms. Paradoxically, the federal government intends to curtail funds for research at a time when many of us believe that we are beginning to understand the basic mechanisms of mental illness.

We have learned that a profession, unlike a craft, cannot be satisfied with customary procedures. We must constantly search for means to organize and to use intelligence in new ways. Obviously, such a search may help us to learn whatever is basic and essential to our task, whatever may be found appropriate and useful to our purpose and to the changing needs of our society. As must be evident, my position, as it has been for many years, is to consider professional education in the tradition of liberal education rather than that of craftsmanship. My hope would be that, whatever changes take place, we will not diminish our basic and fundamental role as clinicians—persons directly and intimately engaged in the study and care of the sick person and his family.

Throughout the centuries, whatever image the physician may have had in the society in which he served, certain qualities have remained transcendent, qualities that made for responsibility, dependability, and accountability; qualities that made possible the compassionate objectivity of the clinician in his care of the sick. In our time as in others, these qualities must be acquired by the psychiatrist as physician.

Bibliography

Brody, E.: Models in psychiatric education. *Journal of Nervous and Mental Disease* 154:153–56, 1972.

44   *American Psychiatry: Past, Present, and Future*

Dain, N.: *Disordered Minds: The First Century of Eastern State Hospital in Williamsburg, Virginia, 1766–1866.* Williamsburg, Va.: The Colonial Williamsburg Foundation, 1971.

Katz, M.: *Current Trends in Mental Health Research: Highlights of the 15th Annual Conference.* Washington, D.C.: Veterans Administration Cooperative Studies in Psychiatry, 1970, pp. 37–39.

Meijering, W. L., and Dekker, E.: Psychiatry and its role in mental health. *Psychiatric Opinion* 10:6–11, 1973.

Redlich, F. C., and Freedman, D. X.: *The Theory and Practice of Psychiatry.* New York and London: Basic Books, 1966, pp. 122.

Romano, J.: The teaching of psychiatry to medical students: Past, present, and future. *American Journal of Psychiatry* 126:1115–26, 1970a.

——: Elimination of the internship—An act of regression. *American Journal of Psychiatry* 126:1565–76, 1970b.

——: The teaching of psychiatry to medical students. *American Journal of Psychiatry* 130:559–62, 1973.

Mainstreams of Therapeutic Modalities

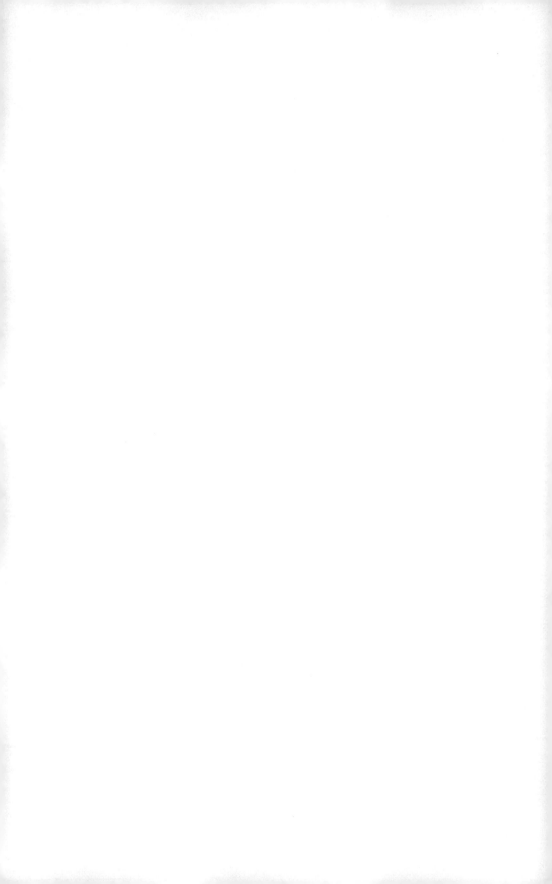

Introduction

James L. Mathis, M.D.

THE rational use of a therapeutic modality in medicine depends upon an understanding of the etiology of the condition to be treated. If the cause of a certain type of highly aberrant behavior were thought to be possession of the body and the mind by malevolent demons, and if these malevolent demons doomed the patient to a future of eternal punishment unless they were exorcized by fire, then the rational treatment of the afflicted patient might be burning at the stake for his own benefit. If the cause of certain types of illnesses manifested by delirium and disorientation or some form of collapse of the mental faculties were known to be an overabundance of blood to the brain, then an obvious rational treatment would be to bleed the patient in order to remove the excess fluids. Each of these treatments has been used in good faith and honest zeal by men of good will, and each was based upon a theory accepted by many of the leading authorities of the day.

There always have been astute thinkers, frequently called skeptics by their friends and heretics by their enemies, who questioned explanations of etiology, and who were not so certain that the accepted therapeutic modalities were based upon adequate proof. Some of the more radical have insisted that unaided human observation was subjective and always attended by possible error. These men have been responsible for changes in etiological theories, and even though some of the changes were retrogressive, a long-term trend of skeptical thinking has been toward a more objective and rational understanding of the functioning of the human and those factors impinging on that functioning.

Today we pride ourselves upon being scientific, and we profess to modify the scientific approach with a laudable degree of humanitarianism. Our scientific advances have answered many questions, but by and large they have raised almost as many as they have put to rest. We, like our ancestors, have changed our therapeutic approach many times to fit the prevailing theory of etiology, and undoubtedly we will do so in the future. Many of us remain skeptical of the present theories, and some of us may even be heretics when certain specific areas are considered.

Most of us in this room would not agree with Weir Mitchell's rest cures nor would we care to endorse a return to the whirling chair and the bleeding knife of Benjamin Rush. On the other hand, some of us who would not espouse these nonscientific approaches to the mentally ill may look with favor upon the treatment of mental conditions by large doses of vitamins, a treatment which may be no more scientifically valid than those of Rush and Mitchell. Even more may use psychotropic drugs in a manner no more rational than ancient trephining of the skull.

Whether or not mental illness as a condition belongs to theology, philosophy, or to medicine remained unsettled for many, many years. The question appeared to be resolved in the 19th century as the treatment of mental illness became a segment of recognized medicine. The search for a specific etiology and therefore for an equally specific treatment intensified. The question of ownership of this massive field of illness did not remain settled for very long. The concept of single etiology did not prove viable, and in the 20th century multiple causation became more and more probable and the theories grew in number and complexity. It followed that each theory produced its more or less specific therapeutic modality, and history began repeating itself as more and more disciplines began to enter the therapeutic arena and to vie for ownership of the mentally ill patient. New disciplines have arisen (and are arising) and the psychiatric field becomes populated with a vast array of new and sometimes instantly produced experts.

The situation may be more advanced, but it is little more stable in 1973 than it was in 1773 or in 1573. We look back upon our predecessors with some degree of admiration mixed with a touch of condescending amusement. We hope sincerely that our followers in this field will look back upon us in a similar length of time with the same degree of both admiration and amusement, but without the condescension. We trust that they will admire us for our honest efforts and open minds, and that they will have improved upon our field of knowledge so much as to be a bit amused at our ignorance. And yet, as we do to those who came before us, we hope that our followers will acknowledge that their improvements will be built upon the painfully laid foundations of the past, however primitive and crude they may appear to them in retrospect.

6. Psychological Approaches

Lawrence C. Kolb, M.D.

AN ANNIVERSARY of an event such as the one we celebrate now in Williamsburg, in commemoration of the bicentennial of the founding of the Eastern State Hospital of Virginia, has importance beyond that of our gathering to do honor to the efforts of our predecessors. It provides an opportunity for review, assessment and reflection upon their efforts and those of their successors up to our own time, an opportunity to reset our course, to rededicate ourselves to the goals of our profession, to sharpen our perspectives so as to identify the significantly new, to broaden our compassion for those caught in the limitations of our struggling efforts of the past and present.

Even before the planning, building, and eventual opening of the institution whose birthday we celebrate today a stirring of change was evident among the more enlightened minds in Western Europe. Coincident with the growing intellectual skepticism and emerging scientific thought of those times, in which the leading thinkers dared to suggest that man had the right to improve his life through the fruitful application of accumulating knowledge, there arose a humanitarian interest in the plight of the so-called lunatic. Two centuries earlier, Weyer had already initiated the challenge to the belief held for so many centuries that mental disturbance was an indication of demonic possession. Within the major institutions of those times the unfortunate victims of mental illness remained chained, massed together, often in filth and exposed like beasts to the curious throng (as in London at Bethlem Hospital), in spite of the earlier pleas of some monastic orders for merciful and tender care for the insane. Evidence of the shift to a recognition that the mentally ill need humanitarian understanding came first when Vincenzio Chiarugi removed the chains from those at Bonifazio Asylum in Florence. Within a decade, in 1793, the second year of the French Revolution, Philippe Pinel struck the chains from the limbs of the manacled sick at the Bicêtre in Paris. By so doing he instituted moral suasion as a therapeutic force by which hospital superintendents and physicians were to control the urge to aggressive violence through respect commanded by their own behavior and voice. Pinel called for public support for an effort to apply to the insane the same humaneness—the rights of liberty and equality—that Marat and Danton demanded for all from the French National Assembly. He thereby laid the ground in the treatment of the mentally ill for acceptance of the humanitarian tenet that man's condition may be improved by man through his own efforts —his own benevolence for mankind.

The moral treatment of the time (Dain 1964) emphasized psychological forces in bringing about behavioral change. It was psychotherapeutic inasmuch as the attitudes and behavior of the caretakers were considered to effect change in the suffering and behavior of the ill. Kindness in meeting the emotional and physical needs of the patient, and respect for his personality, led to change. This treatment was available only to people in the upper and middle socioeconomic classes.

Rush rightly must be seen as the first American physician to undertake serious studies of mental illness. As an individual practitioner he described the thoughts and secrets of his hypothesis and his technical propositions. His perception of the significance of the physician-patient relationship in effecting some "cures" led him to encourage the physician to recognize the importance of a commanding posture. He indicated that many antisocial acts had their origins in emotional disturbance, and recommended gentleness for the depressed, firmness for the manic, and attention-getting actions for the distracted. He also saw a use for threats to induce fear.

The moral therapeutic approach brought remarkable success in terms of patients reported recovered and improved under this regimen from 1800 to mid-century. The statistics show a range of from 48 to 91 percent. Dr. John Galt reported 92 percent recovered at Eastern State Hospital in 1842. Remarkable indeed— such optimistic findings arrived at by putting into practice humanitarian attitudinal change directed by the hospital superintendent to influence staff and patients. It must be recognized, however, that there is little indication of specific individualized methods of treatment such as we know today.

Yet shortly after the founding of our national association in 1846, the record of therapeutic success through moral therapy assumed a progressively downward trend. Was this due to an inability to apply the new attitudinal support or to other forces? Pliny Earle pointed out that the optimistic reporting of earlier years was based on a failure to identify in the reports of success the number of those who recurrently appeared in hospitals as patients in crisis and then recovered sufficiently to return home. Then, too, with the extension of medical care to more people through the zeal of Dorothea Dix, hospitals grew in size and staffing probably became less personal. The nature of the personality problems in the hospital population changed as patients who formerly would have entered the prison system or poorhouses were admitted to mental institutions. But our interest here is not in the vicissitudes of therapeutic valuation but in psychotherapeutic progress. The question before us is perhaps more whether the attitudinal change brought about by skeptical intellectualism of the 18th century, and the accompanying humanitarian attitudes engendered by the political events of those years, constituted the beginnings of psychotherapy or established the ambience in which modern psychotherapy might develop.

There are indeed those who believe today that sociopolitical postures contain within themselves both preventive and psychotherapeutic elements. The psychiatrists of the USSR are the last large and devoted group to become disillusioned by this conviction as they discovered a high national incidence and prevalence of psychosis, which, according to the earlier promises of development of the social man in a communistic state, was expected to disappear, presumably through equality and the relief of economic distress.

This gives rise to the question as to what constitutes psychotherapy. As many of you will recall, Masserman and, later, Kiev, emphasized the similarities of the psychotherapeutic processes used by healers in various cultures over historical time. Jerome Frank (1973) defined the essential elements of psychotherapeutic process as follows: "A series of more or less structured contacts between the healer and the sufferer through which the healer, often with the aid of the group, tries to produce certain changes in the sufferer's emotional state, attitudes and behavior. All concerned believe these changes will help him. Although physical and chemical adjuvants may be used, the healing influence is primarily exercised by works, acts and rituals in which the sufferer, healer and—if there is one—group participate jointly."

That definition points to the need for group support. I would suggest that the sociopolitical scene of those days, which led to the founding of this institution and produced Pinel, Tuke, and others, established the intellectual support for our modern dynamic psychotherapies—psychotherapies which, indeed, differ in many respects from those of the past. And the beginnings of that movement coincided in time with the institutional anniversary we now celebrate. For it was 200 years ago this year that Dr. Anton Mesmer of Vienna first magnetized Fraulein Osterline.

What was unusual about Dr. Mesmer was his attempt to explain the dramatic convulsions he induced by attributing them to the operations of the new science of magnetic or electrical influence. Spoiled by his popularity in Paris, he took on the airs and style of an entertainer. The public display of one wand-wielding man's influence on the behavior of other people was so striking that the French Academy was called on to investigate his work. Commissioners for this investigation included Benjamin Franklin; Lavoisier, the discoverer of oxygen; Guillotin; and others. The commission concluded that "that which has been proven through our examination of magnetism is that man can affect man." The single dissenting member of the commission, de Jussieu, expressed the opinion that in Mesmer's work there might be the nucleus of a psychological idea. In their secret report to Louis XVI the commissioners emphasized the moral dangers of magnetism, pointing out that women were particularly susceptible to its influence. Mesmer was forced to retire but his efforts and his observations had established as a matter of scientific interest the influence of one individual upon another.

Perhaps a lesson can be learned from the charges brought against Mesmer. In psychiatry today we are charged with undermining public morality by our attitudes of patience and concern, and our attempts to understand those who offend socially. Some of the negative pressure currently exerted against our specialty comes from those who perhaps believe that only punitive aversive action can lead to modification of offending behavior. Hypnosis has survived the test of time as a valuable therapeutic technique. It is still used and still taught, and some continue to investigate its psychological parameters. When the Academy of Science investigated "magnetic experiments" again in 1826, a distinguished group which included Magendie, Laënnec, and others affirmed that "magnetism" was a "therapeutic expedient" and had a place in medical science. They recommended that the academy encourage research in the subject seen as a curious branch of psychology and natural history, thus anticipating the beginning of scientific thought about and research into psychotherapy.

But modern psychotherapy as we know it came much later, derived from clinical experimentation and hypothesis. Valuable as it may have been to try to define the essential elements of magical and faith healing of the past and present, and to relate them to similar constituent elements in modern psychotherapy, there are some critical differences. Magic and faith alone are unlikely to achieve the discriminating effort that is based on an understanding of the psychogenetic principles upon which behavioral repertoires are built and against which a psychodynamically appropriate therapeutic approach may be brought to bear. Scientific advance in medicine has come about through progressive evolution of new hypotheses concerning abnormal states of functioning and interventions predicated on that knowledge, tested and retested so as to replicate, refine, or reject the initial hypothesis. This is a different process from the institution of the earlier cures on the basis of hope, faith, or belief.

We must recognize that scientific thinking about psychotherapy came with Sigmund Freud. Another movement concerning behavior, derived largely from animal experimentation, arose at the same time in both Russia and the United States. The origin of learning theory appeared in studies of the conditioned reflexes by I. Pavlov in the USSR and those of Thorndike in the United States and in the early work on operant conditioning. These efforts were not alike, but the methods are not essentially contradictory; the techniques and understanding of each are now on a convergent course influencing one another.

Freud's psychodynamic principles, the tools on which modern American psychotherapy has generally based its foundation, provided a distinguishing feature of the trend within our country. The United States proved more receptive to the psychoanalytic movement than any other nation. The ground was prepared for acceptance here; its proponents were given opportunities consistent with our open (pluralistic) society to explore and to modify the earlier theoretical and traditional propositions put forward in Europe. Teachers of psychoanalytic theory and techniques were welcomed and encouraged to participate in the work of the growing departments of psychiatry of our medical schools and teaching hospitals throughout the land.

In the United States at the turn of the century, Adolf Meyer, unlike most hospital superintendents in this country and abroad, recommended that mental disturbances be recognized as abnormal reactions of men to their human needs, particularly their needs in society. This attitude established the professional frame for acceptance of the new psychotherapies. Meyer's position was later supported by William A. White, superintendent of St. Elizabeth's Hospital. During his training White had been influenced by Boris Sidis, the first psychologist to be appointed to the staff of the New York State Psychiatric Institute in 1896, with whom he conducted experiments on psychological motivation. Curious and analytical, White searched further and, as one might expect in his time, was influenced by psychoanalysis. His breadth, his need to know how to treat and manage patients, stimulated as well a strong interest in sociologic problems related to patient disturbance and hospital treatment. Thus he influenced the teaching and practice of psychotherapeutic medicine.

The great contributions of Meyer and White rest on comprehensive viewpoints which, indeed, distinguish psychiatry in this country today, where they stimulate a willingness to accept the new in psychotherapeutic intervention. Their influence on the great mental hospitals and the clinical facilities attached to the major university medical schools opened the doors to those interested in testing psychoanalytic theory and practice in these settings. It is not surprising that contributions of both Edward J. Kempf and Harry Stack Sullivan flourished with the support of Meyer and White in Baltimore and Washington. Perhaps few modern psychotherapists have reviewed, and probably even fewer have read, that truly remarkable volume on psychopathology by Edward Kempf. Deriving from his deep and intensive studies of patients seen at St. Elizabeth's Hospital in Washington, it presents the first major application of psychoanalytic understanding to the treatment of the schizophrenias in this country. It is required reading even today if one is interested in the psychotherapeutic

approach to such patients. His comprehension of the problem of
transference in the schizophrenias still seems to exceed that of
many modern psychodynamics and many psychotherapists. In his
1924 presidential address before the American Psychiatric Association White states that "since the advent of psychoanalysis we, for
the first time . . . have our interest centered upon the actual
mechanisms that are productive of the symptoms."

There arose at the same time outside of the profession a
freshening interest in the plight of the mentally ill, along with
greater public acceptance of treatment. Clifford Beers, through
his mental hygiene movement, promoted that change in attitude
—and while that movement was not principally concerned with
promoting psychotherapy, it fostered its widespread practice as
the general public learned of the possibilities of change and return to health through psychiatric treatment, in an attitude
optimistic compared with the fears and pessimism of the previous
50 years of hospital care of the mentally ill.

It was our country, then, with its openness, its freedom for
questioning dogmatic positions, its pragmatic attitude and willingness to experiment, that gave the psychoanalytic approach to
psychotherapy its greatest reception and its greatest opportunities.
The groundwork was laid through the teachings and attitudes of
Meyer and White and the introduction of analysis through Put-
nam and Brill. Analysis, too, was influenced by our culture as it
met the emerging social realities of each successive generation.

Some of the older historical writers in psychiatry and analysis
refer to the changes in psychoanalytic theory and technique as
deviations, diversions, or, more mildly, as modifications, suggesting the need to support the beliefs and practices of the psychoanalysis of the immediate past and to make obeisance to its
teachers and leaders. I prefer to consider these changes as
evolutionary strivings, and to see them as shaped by the driving
character of men who pushed eagerly ahead and the pressure of
the clinical material to which they were exposed in their daily
work. The American scene tended to emphasize the social orientation in theory and practice; outcome is more likely to be
measured today in terms of social adaptation. As for the theories
of dynamic psychiatry, interest focused on the social interactions
that lead to distorted personality growth—interactions in the
family and among persons influenced by the values and norms of

the different cultural groups which join together in North America in a more or less common political outlook, and share a common language.

The forward movement in psychotherapy was stimulated by psychoanalytic findings; historians will perhaps see as the most distinctive contribution of North American psychiatrists to this advance the way in which they vigorously pursued a variety of courses. I have referred to Meyer's opening the doors to university departments, mental hospitals, and the new research institutes by his eclecticism. In New York it was possible for Brill to introduce psychoanalysis into the clinical setting of the Vanderbilt Clinic associated with Columbia University, and into the Psychiatric Institute shortly after the turn of this century, with the support of August Hoch. White, along with other mental hospital administrators such as Hutchings, encouraged efforts to apply dynamic principles of treatment in the major mental hospitals. The group therapies, as they appeared in the country's general hospital system, were also influenced relatively quickly by hypotheses stemming from psychoanalytic theory as well as by technical trials in which dynamic teaching was becoming paramount.

Let us examine the medical school. That ground was best prepared perhaps by the extensive teaching of psychiatry to medical students, stimulated by the example set by Adolf Meyer at the new Johns Hopkins Medical School in 1911 and replicated widely throughout the country in succeeding decades. Even professors of medicine became preoccupied with the subject. Walter Palmer at Columbia invited Flanders Dunbar to commence her monumental work on psychosomatic medicine at the Presbyterian Hospital. Schilder studied body image disturbances at Bellevue Hospital. Alexander, Grinker and others influenced the medical faculties at the University of Chicago. These psychiatric explorations, given mostly to etiology, flourished after World War I when the medical students of the prewar era applied their knowledge so extensively in caring for the large number of persons in the armed forces with psychosomatic and psychiatric disabilities. Attempts were made to test brief psychotherapies derived from both the psychobiologic and psychoanalytic models in these hospital situations and to use group therapies with patients in similar disease states to overcome the associated emotional abnormalities. These efforts led to the technical development of brief and focused psychotherapy such as Felix Deutsch's vector analysis, which was devised to direct the therapist's attention to the significant variables in the patient's conflict situation and thus to reduce redundancy and time in treatment. Alexander and his coworkers also suggested modifications in the psychoanalytic approach so as to control and modify behavior by varying the intensity of the transference relationship.

The study and psychotherapeutic management of childhood maladaptations was another major area in which evolution occurred. The first studies in this field were undertaken by Healy in Chicago. Here advance was promoted by the efforts of the National Committee of Mental Hygiene, which, with Commonwealth Fund support, sponsored child guidance clinics and fellowships for study in child psychiatry. Play technique developed as a therapeutic tool, pushed by those who recognized that children using dolls as representatives of important others might associate as freely as adults concerning their conflicted human relations with other people. This projective mechanism provided in a unique way a means of investigating and treating significant fantasies which motivated the disturbing behavior that brought the child to treatment. Many variants on the original play technique have been devised and used since those early days; Redl and others later opened up the way to understand and treat the delinquent child and adolescent.

The psychotherapeutic investigations in the treatment of the psychoses, carried out most extensively by those trained in the Washington-Baltimore area, advanced our knowledge of therapeutic technique as it relates to the sensitive therapist-patient relationship; they also uncovered etiology and invented technical variations more appropriate to the treatment of these forms of psychopathology than those borrowed from and derived from the original psychoanalytic approaches to neurosis. Harry Stack Sullivan will continue to be recognized as the framer of the major concepts used by the talented explorers who gathered together to study first the schizophrenias and, later, the manic depressive reactions. Sullivan, impressed by Meyer and White and perhaps borrowing from Kempf, reached out, in his effort to understand the abstruse communications of his schizophrenic patients, beyond the field of psychopathology to the works of George Mead, the Chicago philosopher, and also to those of Philip Sapir, the linguist.

His efforts fostered the search for new understanding of behavior from the social sciences—a move dictated by the necessities of improving psychotherapeutic theory and technique. Sullivan focused clearly on social experience, commencing with the family, in putting forward his interpersonal theory to account for personality development and its aberrations. He worked to achieve in psychotherapy an understanding by patient and therapist of significant interpersonal events with significant people associated with the inevitable affective arousal and the subsequent personality responses as the source for formation of personality and individual idiosyncrasies. Sullivan also insisted that the therapist recognize himself as a participant observer with responses that would reflect in his patient's behavior; he brought to the psychotherapeutic processes a recognition of the need to study the important variable of the therapist's personality as of scientific and professional importance. His power was in understanding all nuances of communication—verbal and nonverbal—in the determining social expressions and their later emergence in pathological behavior. The conceptual frame developed by him was expanded by detailed studies of others in the Washington group, particularly Frieda Fromm Reichmann, as they related to the treatment of psychoses. In Chicago, Szurek and Adelaide Johnson, influenced by both Alexander and Sullivan in the push toward teaching psychotherapy as a corrective emotional experience in the relation of the patient to the therapist, studied the antisocial acting-out behavior of children and elaborated a powerful hypothesis concerning it. Johnson and others later proposed the need for conjoint therapy of the child with his parents to bring about a change in psychotherapy as well as necessary modification of the psychotherapist's posture in treating certain of the aggressive and sexual perversions.

Some years ago, drawing on the descriptions of variations in psychoanalytic techniques by those just mentioned who concerned themselves with treatment of the psychoses and antisocial acting-out conditions, I enjoyed preparing a paper that detailed, in relation to the known psychopathology of these conditions, the psychotherapeutically useful technical variations from the original analytic technique. Obviously, if the psychodynamics are different, the techniques to bring about behavioral change must also differ.

In her private practice Horney elaborated her concepts of the functional meaning of anxiety beyond those originally derived from Freud's work. She discovered a sense of helplessness in children, a "basic anxiety" which she regarded as a protective device. With her colleagues she came to consider the neuroses as outcomes of conflict between human beings and not simply between the instinctual drives and the environment. She emphasized the need to analyze the character structure of the patient as including unconscious protective devices. To do so, she and others adopted a treatment with greater attention to current conflicts than in the well-established analytic techniques deriving from the European sources. Power, prestige, and aggression were drives that interested her: treatment was more humanized, and value judgments were recognized as inherently necessary in the treatment relationship. Wilhelm Reich's effort to resolve resistances in analytic therapy brought him along similar lines as he focused on the character resistances as protecting armor that maintains the neurotic homeostasis. His concepts made the study and treatment of rigid characters, psychopaths, and so-called borderline psychotics of psychotherapeutic interest. Stimulated by the studies of E. Fromm, Horney, and Kardiner, psychotherapists became more sensitive than before to the influence of cultures on personality development and special character traits.

It is not surprising then that with these new perceptions of the role of social experience in determining behavior, both group and family therapy flourished in this country. As mentioned, group therapy had its beginnings in the medical clinics shortly after the turn of the century, but it was the work of Slavson and others who succeeded him that gave a dynamic theory and understanding to the process. Family therapy, as developed by Ackerman, Don Jackson, and their colleagues, is directly descended from early work with schizophrenic individuals that was influenced by the studies of Sullivan and his colleagues. Today we comprehend the group processes as elaborated by Moreno and, more recently, by Edelson, as providing a sociotherapy—a contribution to ego development and adaptation that goes beyond the goals of individual psychotherapy. Today we see further expression of the group therapies in the many varieties listed by Dr. Romano. Some will survive if they prove helpful in replication. Many are destined to die away as initial enthusiastic hopefulness is followed by inevitable disillusionment.

Behavior therapy, long practiced in the USSR, is among the burgeoning psychotherapeutic efforts of the past decade in this country. It is founded on the premise that all social behaviors are learned, or represent distortions or deficits in the learning process of the developing human; it offers alternative learning processes to replace unsatisfactory learning. These processes either extinguish the early learning that produced the maladaptive behaviors or, where deficits in behavior exist, establish more effective behavioral responses. Such new learning experiences must be associated with the arousal of emotion, either pleasurable as gratification, or painful as aversion. What is striking about the recent work on the behavioral therapies in this country is the growing perception of their resemblance to dynamic therapies in spite of differences, the major one of which is perhaps the emphasis placed in behavior therapy on the control of behavior through "its consequences" rather than its origins in antecedent experiences and repetitive psychodynamically driven response. Thus one must identify ongoing social forces that maintain the unwanted behavior, and eliminate or exclude them to bring about change. To identify one response that induces change the new behavior therapist must examine the role of the relationship of the patient to the therapist as either socially rewarding or aversive, in a way not done before. So, too, the analyst is drawn to a more precise analysis of the rewarding or aversive controls within the continuing social ambience outside the therapeutic hours of each patient he treats. Also, the behaviorist needs to recognize in his patients the often obscure rewards offered by the internal rewarding or aversive systems; this recognition may sometimes come from psychoanalytic insights. But recognition that behavior is maintained and controlled by consequences is indeed influencing the teaching and practice of all forms of psychotherapy, and this emphasis comes from the learning theorists.

Work in the psychotherapeutic field has burgeoned enormously in the past half century, incalculably advancing our knowledge of human relations, our theoretical understanding, and the techniques of approach to the problems of the individual patient. Its advance may well rest with a more open examination and assessment of therapeutic processes now made possible by such modern technologic tools as television, and with scientific scrutiny of outcome in which scientists admit subjective reports of change as well as objective ratings of social adaptation. Health is not necessarily measured for all in the conventional terms of regularly approved social behavior.

Work has proceeded with enthusiasm and vigor in all these areas, although at times without the reflection and control that all new therapeutic techniques must in the long run apply to refine evaluative precision and insure appropriate application. For some, psychotherapy remains today the primary and indicated therapeutic approach; for others, it opens up or supplements the biologic therapeusis. Those with wide knowledge and experience do not overlook the use of the somatic treatments that are so powerful in their capacity to modulate pathological accretions of affect. Many of the younger generation have a broad enough knowledge to encompass a wide span of theory, to know the indications for and against, and to command as well a number of technical variations in applying psychotherapies and combining these therapeutic techniques with the somatic treatments.

In closing, allow me to add to those made earlier my comments on the extraordinary good fortune we have had in this country in federal policies of the last quarter-century which have led to the enlightened development of so many well-trained therapists in the United States. I have recently returned from a country of 20 million which has only 200 psychiatrists, and only two with psychoanalytic training. A young man attending here has told me that in his country of 20 million there is only one psychiatrist!

Bibliography

Braceland, F. J.: *The Institute of Living, The Hartford Retreat, 1822–1972.* Hartford, Conn.: The Institute of Living, 1972.

Bromber, W.: *Man above Humanity; A History of Psychotherapy.* Philadelphia: Lippincott, 1954.

Dain, N.: *Concepts of Insanity in the United States, 1789–1865.* New Brunswick, N.J.: Rutgers University Press, 1964.

Deutsch, A.: *The Mentally Ill in America.* 2d ed. New York: Columbia University Press, 1944.

Frank, J.: *Persuasion and Healing. A Comparative Study of Psychotherapy.* Rev. ed. New York: Johns Hopkins University Press, 1973, pp. 2–3.

Harms, E.: Historical background of psychotherapy as a new scientific field. *Diseases of the Nervous System* 31:116–18, 1970.

Hunt, H.: Behavioural considerations in psychiatric treatment. *Science and Psychoanalysis* 18:36–50, 1971.

Kolb, L. C.: A new look at psychotherapeutic evolution. In *Evolving Concepts in Psychiatry*. Talkington, P. C., and Bloss, C. L. (eds.). New York: Grune & Stratton, 1969.

Rush, B.: *Essays Literary, Moral and Philosophical.* 2d ed. Philadelphia: Bradford, 1806.

Tournay, G.: A history of therapeutic fashions in psychiatry, 1800–1966. *American Journal of Psychiatry* 124:784–96, 1967.

7. Biological Approaches to Treatment and Understanding of the Major Psychoses

Seymour S. Kety, M.D.

B ENJAMIN RUSH, who practiced in my hometown during the period in which the Williamsburg Asylum was established as the first mental hospital in the colonies, had no doubt about the biological origins of mental illness. He treated it with a human centrifuge in the belief that this would improve the circulation of the brain. Although that concept has not been substantiated by modern scientific evidence, his social concerns were among the most thoughtful and articulate of his times. He apparently did not find it necessary to disparage the biological aspects of mental illness in order to recognize and argue for the correction of social ills.

The specificity of the phenothiazines and the butyrophenones against the cardinal symptoms of schizophrenia has recently been recognized. At the same time, it has become clearly established that these agents have an important common action in blocking dopamine receptors in the brain. Conversely, amphetamine potentiates dopamine synapses in the brain, an action that has been shown to be responsible for the stereotyped behavior it induces in animals and one that may well account for other manifestations of schizophrenia, which it induces in man. The tricyclic antidepressants and repeated electroconvulsive shocks appear to potentiate the synaptic activities of biogenic amines, especially norepinephrine and dopamine. A large number of studies in animals have adduced evidence that catecholamine synapses are crucial in the mediation of emotional state, pleasure, and mood. All of these observations have permitted the formulation of heuristic hypotheses of the biological disturbances predisposing to schizophrenia or the affective disorders which can be tested by modern techniques. It is quite possible that from such research

This paper is the revision of an earlier presentation which appears in *Genetics and Psychopathology*, ed. R. Fieve, H. Brill, and D. Rosenthal. Baltimore: The Johns Hopkins Press, 1974.

there may emerge a better understanding of the etiology and pathogenesis of these disorders and the ability to develop more specific and effective therapeutic agents.

My first study of schizophrenia took place just 25 years ago and consisted in applying to that disorder a newly developed technique for measuring the blood flow and energy metabolism of the brain (Kety and Schmidt 1948). Interestingly enough, the development of that technique was aided by a grant from the Scottish Rite Foundation for Research in Dementia Praecox, which was supporting psychiatric research a decade before the National Institute of Mental Health came into existence. Because that foundation had supported our research without questioning its relevance, one of the things we wanted to do once we had this method was to apply it to schizophrenia, since it had been suggested that schizophrenia might be the result of an inadequate circulation to the brain or an insufficiency in its utilization of oxygen. So, with Fritz Freyhan at the Delaware State Hospital and a number of collaborators at the University of Pennsylvania, we undertook a study on a population of 30 schizophrenics displaying various forms of the illness (Kety et al. 1948). We could find no difference from normal in the circulation to the brain or in its oxygen consumption in schizophrenia, and we concluded that it takes just as much oxygen to think an irrational thought as to think a rational one. But, more seriously, we also concluded that if there was a biochemical disturbance in schizophrenia it probably lay in much more subtle and complex processes rather than in the overall circulation and energy metabolism of the brain.

Our knowledge of where to look in the biochemical approach to schizophrenia 25 years ago was just about as meager as that. We had no promising leads; we had no indications of what these more subtle and complex neurochemical processes might be; and without that we could not begin to formulate plausible and heuristic hypotheses.

Eight years later, in the Laboratory of Clinical Science at the National Institute of Mental Health, I had the good fortune to be associated with a remarkable group of colleagues, Axelrod, Evarts, Sokoloff, Kopin, Pollin, Cardon, Kies, and LaBrosse, to mention the names of some of the members of the group. There were a few more hypotheses about schizophrenia at that time, representing bold leaps from rather insufficient basic knowledge to the clinical problem. One hypothesis seemed worth examining. It postulated a defect in the metabolism of circulating epinephrine leading to the accumulation of adrenochrome, a supposedly hallucinogenic metabolite (Hoffer 1957). We quickly realized, however, that we did not know enough about the normal metabolism of epinephrine, let alone its metabolism in schizophrenia. Fortunately, Axelrod was interested in the problem, and, recognizing the importance of the finding of Armstrong and Shaw that a new metabolite, vanillyl-mandelic acid, was excreted in the urine of patients with pheochromocytoma, he laid out, in a short period of time, the metabolic pathways of epinephrine degradation, demonstrated the importance of a new enzyme, catechol-O-methyl-transferase, and characterized the major metabolites (Axelrod 1959). This made it possible for LaBrosse and others of us (1961) to examine the metabolism of circulating epinephrine in schizophrenia. We found no abnormalities and no evidence that the schizophrenic patient made adrenochrome from circulating epinephrine. Axelrod's contributions to fundamental knowledge regarding the catecholamine neurotransmitters have already affected our understanding of the drugs useful in treating the major mental illnesses and have stimulated the development of modern neuropharmacology.

There were many other hypotheses at that time centering upon ceruloplasmin or "taraxein" (which was thought to be a modified form of ceruloplasmin), other plasma proteins, and other putative neurotransmitters, but none of these hypotheses had been confirmed. Thus, in 1959, and again some years later (Kety 1959, 1966), I had to admit that if a young man came to me and asked not for the answer to schizophrenia, not even what the salient biochemical disturbance might be, but simply what aspects of biochemistry he should study if he wanted some day to make a contribution to schizophrenia, I would not have known. I feel differently today. To a considerable extent because of the public support of biomedical, neurobiological, and behavioral research, and the wise philosophy that guided it and its administration, we have learned more about relationships between the brain and behavior in the past 25 years than man had learned in all the previous history of civilization. In contrast to the situation 25 years ago, the remarkable growth of fundamental knowledge now makes very appropriate and promising the development of heuristic hypotheses regarding the etiology of schizophrenia, which can be rigorously tested with techniques that are now available.

There are two current hypotheses which arose from basic research and which seem more capable of tying together observations about schizophrenia and its pharmacology than earlier ones. I should like to indicate some of the reasons why these hypotheses have remained viable and why they are quite promising. There is the transmethylation hypothesis, which was formulated by Harley-Mason (Osmond and Smythies 1952) and which depended upon Cantoni's demonstration of the important biological process of transmethylation. It was suggested that in schizophrenia there is an accumulation of methylated hallucinogenic substances produced in some way by deviant metabolic pathways or by the inability to degrade normal methylated metabolites that would otherwise be rapidly detoxified. Nicotinamide was proposed as a treatment for schizophrenia on the thesis that it was a methyl acceptor and would drain the methyl groups away from the abnormal pathways. Although this vitamin was reported by the original group and has since been regarded as an important treatment for schizophrenia (Hoffer and Osmond 1964), that observation has not been confirmed by more than a dozen controlled studies that have been carried out in this country and in Canada (Lipton et al. 1973). That does not argue against the transmethylation hypothesis, however, since Baldessarini and Kopin showed some years later that nicotinamide did not reduce S-adenosylmethionine in the brain and could hardly compete with transmethylation there.

On the other hand, methionine administration, which tested the hypothesis at another point, on the assumption that it would increase brain levels of S-adenosylmethionine and favor transmethylation, was employed in our laboratory (Pollin, Cardon, and Kety 1961) and in several subsequent studies (Antun et al. 1971), and was found to produce an exacerbation of psychosis in a significant fraction of schizophrenics. Although that was compatible with the transmethylation hypothesis, it could not be taken as evidence in its favor because of the several alternative mechanisms by which methionine could produce a psychotic exacerbation. Nor was it ever conclusively shown that the methionine aggravation is, in fact, an aggravation of the schizophrenic process rather than a toxic or reactive psychosis superimposed upon it.

On the other hand, methionine produces no suggestion of a psychosis in normal volunteers who have received it, and so this finding appears to have more than a tangential relationship to schizophrenia.

Equally interesting is the enzyme first discovered by Axelrod (1961) in the lung, then in the brain by Mandell and Morgan (1971), and confirmed in the brain by Saavedra and Axelrod (1972), capable of methylating normal indoleamines to hallucinogenic substances. Thus, the enzyme will convert tryptamine to dimethyltryptamine, a powerful hallucinogenic substance, and there have been reports that during administration of a methyl-donor, schizophrenic patients who show exacerbation of psychosis also excrete increased quantities of the hallucinogenic dimethyl-tryptamine in their urine (Narasimhachari et al. 1971).

There are also the observations of Friedhoff and Van Winkle (1962) of a methylated congener of dopamine, dimethoxyphenyl-ethylamine, closely related to mescaline, in the urine of schizo-phrenics. Despite considerable controversy this remains a provocative finding that is being explored and extended with appropriate analytical techniques. Its specificity for schizophrenia awaits independent confirmation.

I would like to turn now to a second hypothesis, one that is somehow even more attractive than transmethylation because it can account for more of the schizophrenic syndrome than the presence of hallucinations. The two hypotheses are not necessarily mutually exclusive, and one can speculate about their relationship with each other. The second hypothesis, which is being examined at a number of laboratories, postulates that disturbances in central catecholamine synapses may account for the crucial vulnerability of the schizophrenic and for many of his symptoms. This hypothe-sis is assuming increased importance because of a remarkable series of convergences which strike me as being more than coincidences.

Much more than LSD or any of the hallucinogens, amphetamine has the ability to produce in most individuals who receive it in sufficient doses a toxic psychosis difficult to distinguish from a paranoid schizophrenic reaction. For this we have the most recent testimony of a group (Angrist and Gershon 1971) that has studied this phenomenon extensively. It is interesting that amphetamine has a number of actions, but most of these actions involve the catecholamine system in the brain. Amphetamine releases dopamine and norepinephrine at catecholamine-containing nerve endings, and in other ways potentiates the action of these putative transmitters at their synapses in the brain (Glowinski and Axelrod 1965). Here we have the first convergence: amphetamine psychosis (which resembles schizophrenia) may be produced by an activation of catecholamine synapses in the brain. More recently, we have had the stimulating neuropharmacological work of Snyder and his colleagues (Snyder et al. 1970; Taylor and Snyder 1971) and the studies of Randrup and Munkvad (1970) to suggest that the psychosis and the stereotyped behavior which is produced by amphetamine in man or animals is likely to be related to its effect at dopamine rather than norepinephrine receptors.

There is also the independent body of knowledge stemming from the discovery of chlorpromazine and the succeeding antipsychotic drugs and dealing with their mechanism of action. There was first the important clinical observation that both the phenothiazines and the butyrophenones, which were discovered by serendipity and quite independently, are both effective against schizophrenia although they are not related chemically, and both produce symptoms of Parkinson's disease as important side effects. I remember the clinicians who were among the first to use the phenothiazines 15 to 20 years ago saying that unless one got the beginning of Parkinsonian symptoms, one was probably not giving enough of the drug to produce the greatest therapeutic benefit in schizophrenia.

That important observation became the source of some heuristic speculation about schizophrenia once our body of fundamental information permitted a better understanding of Parkinson's disease. That, in turn, required the discovery of the fluorescent properties of certain catecholamine-conjugated products, the development of suitable histofluorescent techniques, their application to the brain (Hillarp, Fuxe, and Dahlström 1966), the identification of a dopamine-containing nigrostriatal pathway (Anden et al. 1966), and eventually the demonstration (Hornykiewicz 1963) that Parkinson's disease was associated with a deficiency of dopamine in the striatum. That information, coupled with the accumulated knowledge of the biosynthesis of dopamine, led to the effective treatment of Parkinson's disease with L-dopa. It also led to an understanding of the mechanism of action of the antipsychotic drugs and, perhaps, to an elucidation of some of the biological processes at fault in schizophrenia.

In 1963, Carlsson suggested that the phenothiazines produced a blockade of dopamine receptors in the brain. Several laboratories have now (Carlsson and Lindqvist 1963; Anden, Roos, and Verdinius 1964; Nybäck, Borzecki, and Sedvall, 1968) adduced evidence that this was so for the phenothiazines and butyrophenones, although the explanation of their therapeutic effects is still incomplete (Matthysse 1973).

Meanwhile, more clinical information was being acquired about the therapeutic effects of these drugs, which were at first thought to be merely "chemical strait jackets" that suppressed aggressive or disturbed behavior. Davis (1965), examining the results of a large number of double-blind studies on the phenothiazine drugs in schizophrenia, noted that the most prominent effect of these drugs was upon the cardinal features of schizophrenia as they were described by Kraepelin (i.e., on thought disorder, blunted affect, withdrawal, and autistic behavior); this suggests that these drugs are providing more than symptomatic relief, that they may, in fact, be acting more specifically on biological processes in schizophrenia.

Thus we have seen in the past 10 years a series of interesting clinical observations and an accumulation of basic information converging on the activity of dopamine and certain of its synapses in the brain to explain both the psychotic, stereotyped behavior induced by amphetamine and the antipsychotic therapeutic effects of the phenothiazines and butyrophenones. This has suggested to more than one observer that dopamine and its pathways in the brain must play a special role in schizophrenia. In fact, the alternative to that inference is that it is a series of coincidences that apomorphine, which produces stereotyped behavior, and the amphetamines, which stimulate schizophrenia, also stimulate dopamine receptors in the brain, while the phenothiazines and butyrophenones, discovered independently to have important therapeutic effects in schizophrenia and to prevent drug-induced stereotypy, also block dopamine receptors.

Although I feel that these observations are unlikely to be mere coincidences and that dopamine must be playing an important role in schizophrenia, I also feel that dopamine is only part of the story. We must avoid premature closure and keep our thinking open to other neurotransmitters and additional pathways which may be involved. Thus, one may account for the stereotyped behavior of schizophrenia on the basis of increased activity of dopamine receptors, but there are other features of schizophrenia responsive to the antipsychotic drugs which no known action on dopamine receptors can explain. I am thinking of the flatness of affect, the anhedonia, withdrawal, and autism of schizophrenia. Some of these manifestations are suggestive of behavioral changes produced in animals by depletion or blockade of norepinephrine.

We are far from understanding the precise behavioral role of that transmitter at its central synapses, but there is considerable evidence to support its involvement in the mediation of exploratory and affective behavior, in motivation, and in mood (Segal and Mandell 1970; Stein 1964; Slangen and Miller 1969; Redmond et al. 1971). Monkeys which have received alpha-methyl-paratyrosine, which quite specifically blocks catecholamine synapses, make fairly good animal models of the withdrawal, absence of affect, lack of motivation, and even catatonia of the schizophrenic.

It would seem that a defect which would result in an overactivity of dopamine and an underactivity of norepinephrine would account for more of the manifestations of schizophrenia than a change in dopamine activity alone. This focuses our attention immediately on dopamine-beta-hydroxylase (DBH), the enzyme responsible for the conversion of dopamine to norepinephrine. Is it possible that this enzyme operates as a switch in altering the ratio of dopamine to norepinephrine which is produced at certain synapses?

There is a precedent for such an enzyme effect, which was discovered by Wurtman and Axelrod (1966), involving an enzyme in the adrenal medulla, phenylethanolamine-N-methyltransferase, which converts norepinephrine to epinephrine. This enzyme appears to play an important role in regulating the ratio of epinephrine to norepinephrine which is secreted by that gland; and, interestingly enough, the corticosteroids secreted by the adrenal cortex and passing by way of a special portal circulation to the medulla are able to affect the ratio of these two catecholamines by action on the enzyme. Now, in DBH were playing a similar role in the brain, regulating the ratio of norepinephrine to dopamine, a defect in that enzyme or its regulation could produce the alteration in that ratio which is suggested by the manifestations of schizophrenia. Thoenen and associates (1965) have shown that at a peripheral noradrenergic synapse, dopamine is released in perceptible amount if DBH is inhibited. It is not impossible that noradrenergic endings in the brain are capable of releasing dopamine or norepinephrine, transmitters with different effects, their ratio depending on the DBH activity there and the factors which affect it.

There are some observations on schizophrenia which are compatible with that notion. Antabuse has been reported to produce a psychotic reaction in some schizophrenics who receive it (Heath et al. 1965). Dopamine-beta-hydroxylase is one of the enzymes that are inhibited by antabuse. Although L-dopa in large doses can produce psychotic side effects, one group has reported that, given in moderate dosage to schizophrenics who are being treated with phenothiazines, it significantly enhanced the therapeutic effect (Inanoga et al. 1972). Since the phenothiazine blockade of dopamine receptors is much greater than that on norepinephrine receptors (Neff and Costa 1966), L-dopa administration could result in greater norepinephrine effects if given in conjunction with phenothiazines. The latter drugs, per se, may enhance norepinephrine effects by stimulating catecholamine synthesis via a feedback mechanism activated by a blockade of dopamine receptors but leaving the norepinephrine receptors relatively free to respond to the increased norepinephrine. Pimozide, a new antipsychotic agent which blocks only dopamine receptors, increases mood and motivation in chronic schizophrenics. This hypothetical mechanism would help to explain such effects.

The most recent and interesting observation pertinent to this hypothesis was made by Wise and Stein (1973), who found post mortem a 40 percent reduction in DBH activity in the brains of schizophrenics as compared to nonschizophrenic controls. A large number of artifacts can occur in such studies, and these authors were aware of and took great pains to rule out the effects of age, post mortem degradation, and chronic phenothiazine administration. Should this observation be confirmed, it could be for schizophrenia what Hornykiewicz's finding was for Parkinson's disease. Another very compelling and well-controlled finding which is free of the difficulties inherent in post mortem studies is the observation by Wyatt and his collaborators (1973) at the National Institute of Mental Health, that monoamine oxidase is significantly reduced in the platelets of schizophrenics, and equally in the schizophrenic and nonschizophrenic members of monozygotic twin pairs discordant for schizophrenia. The authors suggest that monoamine oxidase may be a genetic marker for schizophrenia. If the reduction in monoamine oxidase also occurs in the brain it could result in various disturbances in central amine metabolism, including increased dopamine and serotonin activity or the accumulation of hypothetical methylated and hallucinogenic amines.

It is clearly too early to put all of these observations together into a single definitive hypothesis that would "explain" schizophrenia. Nevertheless, I have the feeling, which I have never had before, that we are beginning to see the light at the end of the tunnel. There are powerful new techniques, such as mass fragmentography, more specific pharmacological agents, precursors, and enzyme inhibitors. There are new immunochemical techniques for identifying and assaying enzymes and specifying their regional localization (Hartman, Zide, and Udenfriend 1972). There are the techniques of cell culture and the ingenious endocrine window which Sachar has opened (Sachar et al. 1971) for inferring aminergic activity in the human brain from hypothalamically released endocrine responses.

Recent genetic evidence (Kety et al. 1968, 1974) gives ample testimony that schizophrenia is more than a myth and provides a strong justification for seeking the biological processes required for the expression of the genetic components which are clearly involved in schizophrenic illness. Moreover, in contrast to the situation one or two decades ago, we now have some fair idea of where to look for the biological substrates on which life experience builds. The foundations which the National Institute of Mental Health helped to build up during the past 25 years now appear to be capable of bearing weight. The store of fundamental information acquired during that time provides the basis for a number of heuristic and plausible hypotheses which do not attempt to solve the problem all at once but indicate important stepping stones to that goal. We can also see large areas of behavior and biology which remain to be further elucidated and joined. During that time, research has become a powerful ally of psychiatry (Kety 1961), substituting inquiry for dogma, scientific examination for impressionistic thinking. A cohort of psychiatrists has been trained and has become skilled in clinical investigation and fundamental research. Never has the time been more propitious or progress been more promising. We can assure that progress by a prudent distribution of our resources, by investing more than a fraction of 1 percent of the cost of mental illness in clinical and basic research, and in continued research training. This we will do if we are not hampered by a penny-wise, pound-foolish fiscal policy, or misled by those who would solve the problem of mental illness by denying its existence.

Bibliography

Anden, N. E., Fuxe, K., Hamberger, B., and Hökfelt, T.: A quantitative study on the nigro-neostriatal dopamine neuron system in rats. *Acta Physiologica Scandinavica* 67:306–12, 1966.

Anden, N. E., Roos, B. E., and Verdinius, B.: Effects of chlorpromazine, haloperidol and reserpine on the level of phenolic acids in the rabbit corpus striatum. *Life Science* 3:149–58, 1964.

Angrist, B. M., and Gershon, S.: A pilot study of pathogenic mechanisms in amphetamine psychosis utilizing differential effects of D- and L-amphetamine. *Pharmakopsychiatrie* 4:64–75, 1971.

Antun, F. T., Burnett, G. B., Cooper, A. J., Daly, R. J., Smythies, J. R., and Zealley, A. K.: The effects of l-methionine (without MAOI) in schizophrenia. *Journal of Psychiatric Research* 8:63–71, 1971.

Axelrod, J.: The metabolism of catecholamines *in vivo* and *in vitro*. *Pharmacological Reviews* 11:402–8, 1959.

——: Enzymatic formation of psychotomimetic metabolites from normally occurring compounds. *Science* 134:343–44, 1961.

Baldessarini, R. J., and Kopin, I.: S-adenosylmethionine in brain and other tissues. *Journal of Neurochemistry* 13:764–77, 1966.

Carlsson, A., and Lindqvist, M.: Effect of chlorpromazine or haloperidol on formation of 3-methoxytyramine and normetanephrine in mouse brain. *Acta Pharmacologica et Toxicologica* 20:140–44, 1963.

Davis, J. M.: Efficacy of the tranquilizing and antidepressant drugs. *Archives of General Psychiatry* 13:552–72, 1965.

Friedhoff, A. J., and Van Winkle, E.: Characteristics of an amine found in urine of schizophrenic patients. *Journal of Nervous and Mental Diseases* 135:550–55, 1965.

Glowinski, J., and Axelrod, J.: Effects of drugs on the uptake, release and metabolism of H^3-norepinephrine in the rat brain. *Journal of Pharmacology and Experimental Therapeutics* 149:43–49, 1965.

Hartman, B. K., Zide, D., and Udenfriend, S.: The use of dopamine-beta-hydroxylase as a marker for the central noradrenergic system in rat brain. *Proceedings of the National Academy of Science (U.S.A.)* 69:2722–26, 1972.

Heath, R. G., Nesselhof, W., Bishop, M. P., and Byers, L. N.: Behavioral and metabolic changes associated with administration of tetra-ethylthiuram disulfide (antabuse). *Diseases of the Nervous System* 26:99–105, 1965.

Hillarp, N. E., Fuxe, K., and Dahlström, A.: Demonstration and mapping of central neurons containing dopamine, noradrenaline, and 5-hydroxytryptamine and their reactions to psychopharmaca. *Pharmacological Reviews* 18:727–41, 1966.

Hoffer, A.: Epinephrine derivatives as potential schizophrenic factors. *Journal of Clinical and Experimental Psychopathology* 18:27, 1957.

——, and Osmond, H.: Treatment of schizophrenia with nicotinic acid. *Acta Psychiatrica Scandinavica* 40:171–89, 1964.

Hornykiewicz, O.: Die topische lokalisation und das verhalten von noradrenalin und dopamin in der substantia negra des normalen und Parkinson-kranken menschen. *Wiener Klinische Wochenschrift* 75:309–12, 1963.

Inanoga, K., Inoue, K., Tachibana, H., Oshima, M., and Kotorii, T.: Effect of L-dopa in schizophrenia. *Folia Psychiatrica et Neurologica Japonica* 26:145–57, 1972.

Kety, S. S.: Biochemical theories of schizophrenia. A two-part critical review of current theories and of the evidence used to support them. *Science* 129:1528–32, 1959.

——: The Academic Lecture: The heuristic aspect of psychiatry. *American Journal of Psychiatry* 118:385–97, 1961.

——: Current biochemical research in schizophrenia. In *Psychopathology of Schizophrenia*. Hoch, P. H., and Zubin, J. (eds.). New York: Grune & Stratton, 1966, pp. 225–32.

——, and Schmidt, C. F.: Nitrous oxide method for a quantitative determination of cerebral blood flow in man: Theory, procedure and normal values. *Journal of Clinical Investigation* 27:476–83, 1948.

——, Woodford, R. B., Harmel, M. H., Freyhan, F. A., Appel, K. E., and Schmidt, C. F.: Cerebral blood flow and metabolism in schizophrenia. The effects of barbiturate semi-narcosis, insulin coma and electroshock. *American Journal of Psychiatry* 104:765–70, 1948.

——, and Matthysse, S. (eds.): Prospects for research on schizophrenia. *Neurosciences Research Programs Bulletin* 10:449–95, 1972.

——, Rosenthal, D., Wender, P. H., and Schulsinger, F.: The types and prevalence of mental illness in the biological and adoptive families of adopted schizophrenics. In *The Transmission of Schizophrenia*. Rosenthal, D., and Kety, S. S. (eds.). Oxford: Pergamon Press, 1968, pp. 345–62.

——, Rosenthal, D., Wender, P. H., Schulsinger, F., and Jacobsen, B.: Mental illness in the biological and adoptive families of adopted individuals who have become schizophrenic: A preliminary report based upon psychiatric interviews. In *Genetics and Psychopathology,* Fieve, R., Brill, H., and Rosenthal, D. (eds.). Baltimore: Johns Hopkins University Press, 1974.

LaBrosse, E. H., Mann, J. D., and Kety, S. S.: The physiological and psychological effects of intravenously administered epinephrine and its metabolism in normal and schizophrenic men. III Metabolism of 7-H³-epinephrine as determined in studies on blood and urine. *Journal of Psychiatric Research* 1:68–75, 1961.

Lipton, M. E., Ban, T. A., Kane, F. J., Levine, J., Mosher, L. R., and Wittenborn, R.: *Report of the American Psychiatric Association Task Force on Vitamin Therapy and Psychiatry.* Washington: American Psychiatric Association, 1973.

Mandell, A. J., and Morgan, M.: Indole (ethyl) amine N-methyl-transferase in human brain. *Nature; New Biology* 230:85–87, 1971.

Matthysse, S.: The state of the evidence. In *Proceedings of the Symposium on Catecholamines and Their Enzymes in the Neuropathology of Schizophrenia.* Kety, S. S., and and Matthysse, S. (eds.). London: Pergamon Press, 1973.

Narasimhachari, N., Heller, B., Spaide, J., Haskovec, L., Fujimori, M., Tabushi, K., and Himwich, H. E.: Urinary studies of schizophrenics and controls. *Biological Psychiatry* 3:9–20, 1971.

Neff, N. H., and Costa, E.: Effect of tricyclic antidepressants and chlorpromazine on brain catecholamine synthesis. *Proceedings of the 1st International Symposium on Antidepressant Drugs.* Excerpta Medica International Congress Series no. 122: Milan, 1966, pp. 28–34.

Nybäck, H., Borzecki, Z., and Sedvall, G.: Accumulation and disappearance of catecholamines formed from tyrosine-¹⁴C in mouse brain. *European Journal of Pharmacology* 4:395–403, 1968.

Osmond, H., and Smythies, J.: Schizophrenia: A new approach. *Journal of Mental Science* 98:309–15, 1952.

Pollin, W., Cardon, P. V., and Kety, S. S.: Effects of amino acid feedings in schizophrenic patients treated with iproniazid. *Science* 133:104–5, 1961.

Randrup, A., and Munkvad, I.: Biochemical, anatomical and psychological investigations of stereotyped behavior induced by amphetamines. In *Amphetamines and Related Compounds.* Costa, E., and Garattinis, S. (eds.). New York: Raven Press, 1970.

Redmond, D. E., Maas, J. W., Kling, A., and Dekirmenjean, H.: Changes in primate social behavior after treatment with alpha-methyl-paratyrosine. *Psychosomatic Medicine* 33:97–113, 1971.

Saavedra, J. M., and Axelrod, J.: Psychotomimetic N-methylated tryptamines: Formation in brain *in vivo* and *in vitro. Science* 175:1365, 1972.

Sachar, E. J., Finkelstein, J., and Hellman, L.: Growth hormone and responses in depressive illness: Response to insulin tolerance test. *Archives of General Psychiatry* 24:263–64, 1971.

Segal, D. S., and Mandell, A. J.: Behavioral activation of rats during intraventricular infusion of norepinephrine. *Proceedings of the National Academy of Sciences (U.S.A.)* 66:289–93, 1970.

Slangen, J. L., and Miller, N. E.: Pharmacological tests for the function of hypothalamic norepinephrine in eating behavior. *Physiology and Behavior* 4:543–52, 1969.

Snyder, S. H.: Catecholamines in the brain as mediators of amphetamine psychosis. *Archives of General Psychiatry* 27:169–79, 1972.

Stein, L.: Self-stimulation of the brain and the central stimulant action of amphetamine. *Federation Proceedings* 23:836–50, 1964.

Taylor, K. M., and Snyder, S. H.: Differential effects of d- and l-amphetamine on behavior and on catecholamine in dopamine and norepinephrine containing neurons of rat brain. *Brain Research* 28:295–309, 1971.

Thoenen, H., Haefely, W., Gey, K. F., and Hürlimann, A.: Diminished effects of sympathetic nerve stimulation in cats pretreated with disulfiram: Liberation of dopamine as sympathetic transmitter. *Life Sciences* 4:2033–38, 1965.

Thudichum, J. L. W.: *A Treatise on the Chemical Constitution of the Brain Based Throughout upon Original Researches.* London: Bailliere, Tindall & Cox, 1884.

Wise, C. D., and Stein, L.: Dopamine-beta-hydroxylase deficits in the brains of schizophrenic patients. *Science* 181:344–47, 1973.

Wurtman, R. J., and Axelrod, J.: Control of enzymatic synthesis of adrenaline in the adrenal medulla by adrenal cortical steroids. *Journal of Biological Chemistry* 241:2301–5, 1966.

Wyatt, R. J., Murphy, D. L., Belmaker, R., Donnelly, C., Cohen, S., and Pollin, W.: Reduced monoamine oxidase activity in platelets: A possible genetic marker for vulnerability to schizophrenia. *Science* 179:916–18, 1973.

8. Social-Community Approaches in Psychiatry

Melvin Sabshin, M.D.

Introduction

THE *uniqueness* of a bicentennial commemoration of an American psychiatric institution provides a superb occasion for reminiscing, for reviewing, and for anticipating the future. I was delighted to be asked to be a participant in this special program, and I have a new reason for delight. Two years ago when I accepted the invitation I did not have the slightest glimmer about the possibility of becoming the next Medical Director of the APA, and my comments today represent my *first* opportunity to make a presentation subsequent to official action on this appointment by the APA Board of Trustees. I am grateful to those kind fates and to my friends here for permitting me to arrange my initial presentation after the appointment in such an auspicious context. I am certain that you will understand that the long and illustrious history of the APA becomes inextricably intertwined in my mind at this moment with the great beginnings here in Williamsburg 71 years before the medical superintendents, including two Virginians, formed their new association in 1844—an association which ultimately became the APA.

There is something quite significant about the early period of psychiatry in the United States which not only pertains to the historic occasion that we commemorate today but is also quite relevant to the specific topic I am to discuss. The era of "moral treatment" in American psychiatry that Bockhoven (1963) has described so aptly, and which Professor Dain elaborated upon yesterday, began in the wake of our revolutionary war, and this era was indeed one of the most progressive and exciting periods in the history of psychiatry. Many humanitarian social movements were initiated and propelled by the American Revolution and its sequelae. I realize that as a non-Virginian I am bringing coals to Williamsburg and to Monticello (if not Newcastle) to speak about this subject in the shadow of the brilliant and courageous Virginians whose leadership was so indispensable to all of those events—within psychiatry and for the Revolution itself. Nevertheless I wish to remind this audience and others who may read these remarks that the pioneers of American psychiatry were indeed engaged in a great experiment of utilizing social techniques for the care of psychiatric patients. In retrospect it appears clear that the social-community approaches were the major positive therapeutic modalities available to the superintendents and their staffs at the psychiatric hospitals of the late 1700s and the early 1800s. The superintendents understood very well that sustained kindness and humanitarian care provided in a particular setting were vital factors in the recovery from mental illness. They practiced what they philosophized about and, as illustrated by Pliny Earle's 50-year follow-up study, their results were excellent, including a rehospitalization rate reported to be lower than what we subsequently achieved.

Indeed, in this latter third of the 20th century we are still searching for that early enlightened spirit. It grew dim with the massive waves of immigration during the late 19th century, the rapid increase in our population, the growth and proliferation of urbanization, and the lugubrious pessimism dominating the psychiatric world in the latter part of the 19th century and the first part of this century. We began to recover some of the optimistic humanism with the mental hygiene and child guidance movements that came after the First World War, but the motivation and the light dimmed quickly in the face of inadequate resources in the turmoil of our economic depression and the subsequent Second World War. The same irrepressible forces emerged again in the 1960s; we have now approached the point of deciding whether or not the social-community developments of the 1960s will endure with a broadened base and a more innovative style or recede, only to return again in another cycle. Most of my comments today will deal with the events of this more recent ebb and flow, the currents that shaped them, and what they might portend for the future.

Definition of Social Psychiatry and Its Applications

At this point I should like to change the style and tempo of the presentation by confronting just what I mean by the subject of this paper—namely, the social-community approaches in psychiatry. As I anticipated, my predecessors on the platform today have utilized a multivariate, or at least a pluralistic approach. Both Drs. Kolb and Kety have included *social* or *environmental* or *cultural* variables in their discussion, as is certainly appropriate in dealing with a plethora of clinical problems in which causality and intervening mechanisms are still being explored.

In previous attempts to define social psychiatry (Sabshin 1966a, 1966b) I emphasized its emergence as an increasingly coherent group of middle-level theories subsumed under the sociobehavioral sciences. These theories involve sophisticated utilization of *independent* social variables to predict and to explain a series of *dependent* psychiatric variables. Furthermore, social psychiatry involves the rational employment of *independent* social variables as general and particular modalities to alter *dependent* psychiatric variables.

Thus this concept of social psychiatry involves etiological systems, therapeutic approaches, and those variables intervening with the proviso that the social factors are conceived as the *independent* variables. By discussing the social variables as independent in this context the emphasis is upon those social factors that might be the determinants or codeterminants of psychiatric syndromes, e.g., the social isolation *hypothesis* and schizophrenia. This definition of social psychiatry essentially excludes the reverse impact of independent psychiatric variables upon social systems, e.g., the impact of a significant number of retardates on a particular society—or the impact of large numbers of discharged mental patients on a particular community. Fascinating as those questions are, I believe that they fall outside the sphere of social psychiatry.

From the treatment modality perspective, the social approaches also involve the employment of independent social variables in the therapeutic process. Thus the development and maintenance of a threapeutic milieu is an example of a social approach. Of course, such a milieu induces *psychological* changes in individual patients and may even alter biological systems; those effects are dependent outflows from the social variables.

There is, of course, the age-old problem of distinguishing *social* from *psychological* independent variables. At the extremes we can achieve reasonable consensus (e.g., intrapsychic variables fall under the psychological rubric and the impact of social class appears to transcend psychological variation in many areas). At the borderland we can debate to what extent dyadic relationships or family interactions or group processes represent social as compared to psychological approaches. Since I do not believe that territoriality is the major question for this presentation, I will not pursue this point; I simply wish to remind you of its presence and its importance.

After defining or delimiting the term *social* for this presentation it is important to note that treatment systems represent the application of social psychiatric concepts to a variety of pragmatic settings. In this context community psychiatry is one of the major action subsets of social psychiatry. A number of other psychiatric sectors are part of the action systems in transaction with social psychiatric variables. Much hospital psychiatry falls under this rubric, as does a large portion of adolescent, child, and geriatric psychiatry. The sectors also include much of forensic psychiatry, military psychiatry, industrial psychiatry, student health psychiatry, orthopsychiatry, preventive psychiatry (especially primary prevention), public health psychiatry, transcultural psychiatry, ethnopsychiatry, family psychiatry, religion and psychiatry, group psychotherapy, and a variety of other related fields, including ecopsychiatry (ecology and psychiatry). It is clear that there is no limit to the number of adjectives that can be and have been placed before the word *psychiatry,* and we shall ride in all directions with multiple terminology until a new synthesis can be achieved.

Obviously there is marked overlap among the sectors mentioned above, but they can be classified under three major rubrics. One involves geographic, spatial, or organizational entities—e.g., hospital psychiatry. A second involves developmental systems with age-specific adaptational tasks in which knowledge of the social context variables affecting that age group is vital in the understanding of psychiatric problems common to the age group. Indeed, it would be very hard to deal therapeutically with psychological problems of older people without an awareness of the adaptive tasks and problems of the elderly in a particular society. A third subset among the various sectors involves a group of functional therapeutic processes such as special communication networks—for example, that occurring in group psychotherapy or in family therapy. Each sector involves an action system, or, if you will, a therapeutic modality, but no sector should be considered simply as an applied field *unless* one clearly includes within a definition of applied field the probability that the central body of theory is constantly affected by the application. Of course, there is pluralism in each of these areas and an overlap with psychological and biological levels. Various combinations exist. Sociobiology, for example, involves the conjoint effect of social and biological variables upon behavioral phenomena.

Recent History of Social Psychiatry

At this stage I would like to review and to summarize some of the forces which converged into the social-community approaches of the past decade.

Harry Stack Sullivan (1931) provided major impetus to social psychiatry as it has evolved in the United States. In the early 1920s there were lively debates and exchanges of ideas between Sullivan, Sapir, and Elliott. Indeed, these discussions were concerned with concepts which are equally relevant a half century later. The mental hygiene movement in the United States did not specifically ally itself to social psychiatric concepts, but it was definitely related to the ameliorative social psychiatric movements simultaneously developing in Germany and in England (Dreikurs 1961). The movement died in Germany with Hitler's rise, but, quite significantly, West Germany became one of the world's major social psychiatric centers during the past decade (Dörner and Plog 1972).

Transcultural psychiatry and the field of culture and personality have had vicissitudes pertinent to the evolution of social psychiatry. During the 1940s there was a flowering of interdisciplinary work among anthropologists, psychiatrists, and psychoanalysts. The influence of Boaz, Mead, and Benedict upon psychiatrists was at a peak, and there were widespread repercussions of this exchange across disciplinary lines. Abram Kardiner's (1939) ideas typified progressive applications of anthropology to the mental health field. Kardiner's ideas, among other things, influenced many of us who entered psychiatry during the late 1940s. In working with Linton, Kardiner attempted to formulate a theory of basic personality structure for specific societies, and his work on relatively primitive subsystems was quite exciting to many of us in the breadth and scope of its explanatory powers. When he attempted to apply the same model to American small-town urban society, however, he had great difficulty, and his work was criticized as being too global and inappropriate for the complex changing urban culture. When Kardiner engaged in an analysis of a particular American subculture in his study of the American black (1951) there was even more criticism, and, sad to say, his work is much less visible to a whole new generation of psychiatrists. In my opinion, the apparent decline of Kardiner's influence on psychiatrists and psychoanalysts was symbolic of a lessening of what had been during the period 1950 to 1965 a more than casual interest of psychiatrists in the field of culture and personality.

For *psychiatrists,* the social psychiatry of the 1950s and early 1960s filled in to some extent a vacuum left by the decline of serious interest in culture and personality. Since 1965, however, there has been a revival of interest in transcultural psychiatry. This spurt has been stimulated in part by the growth of psychiatry in Africa, Asia, and South America, and the growing communication and travel across continental and national boundaries. WHO, the World Federation of Mental Health, and the National Institute of Mental Health have facilitated this trend by fostering crossnational comparative studies (Kramer 1969). At the May 1973 meeting of the APA in Honolulu the dominant theme of the meeting involved transcultural psychiatry; I was particularly impressed with the freshness of ideas and the increased awareness of the theoretical yield that might be obtained by a new merger of social with transcultural psychiatry. Talented psychiatrists working with colleagues in anthropology, sociology, and social psychology are beginning to resume serious investigative work—and this is a most promising area for the future.

Another major force catalyzing interest in social approaches has arisen in the arena of psychiatric epidemiology. Growing out of the public health tradition and heavily influenced by models of physical illness, epidemiology has attracted a small but articulate group of psychiatrists and other behavioral scientists. By and large, however, it has been virtually ignored by most of the psychiatric profession. In part, this reaction relates to a number of conceptual and methodological problems which still beset our field. In my judgment, an insufficiently acknowledged ambiguity in the fundamental distinctions between mental health and mental illness is a major stumbling block. In our book on normality (Offer and Sabshin 1966), Offer and I have cited and illustrated the widely diverging perspectives on normality and health still extant. These variances in basic definitions have among other consequences plagued our epidemiology and have lead to blind alleys such as those studies using a "utopian" concept of health which report a very high incidence and prevalence of mental disease. If health is conceptualized as an ideal state which can be only approximated in real life, everybody is to some extent ill. In our book, Offer and I made a special plea for empirical research on healthy populations to replace the traditional deductive generalizations with longitudinal studies on healthy populations. A review of the past decade shows a promising trend toward such empirical normative studies (Offer and Sabshin, 1974; Holmstrom 1972) and gives hope that comparative analysis of these diverse groups may lead to new hypotheses and theories of mental illness as well as new formulations of adaptive behavior. One interesting finding is that an overwhelming number of such studies of healthy populations have involved white middle-class male populations. Women's groups and minorities have more than a modicum of truth in their assertion that they tend to be falsely viewed as vulnerable, sick, and deviant when they are compared with normative models derived from other populations. Returning to epidemiology per se, it is my belief that the lack of empirically derived normative data has inhibited the full development of a scientific epidemiology (other than that based on *gross* signs of psychopathology).

Other forces germane to the social psychiatric arena reflect a quarter of a century of work in human transactions transcending individual psychology. Studies of familial interaction, group processes, marital adaptation, etc., have taken hold with intermittent and variable achievements. In part, this movement demonstrated the impact of transactional human processes upon individual pathology and pari passu raised serious questions regarding many concepts of human behavior formulated primarily out of intrapsychic or solely intraindividual data. A particularly disturbing recent trend, however, relates to the efflorescence of therapies which appear to assume a strikingly anti-intellectual and antiscientific attitude. Certain segments of the encounter group movement illustrate this tendency and, as has been pointed out by several observers, its rapid growth in the United States reflects a variety of societal tensions. Unfortunately, recent trends have discouraged a number of researchers from entering the field, and the scientific output has been seriously retarded (Yalom et al. 1970).

Social psychiatry has also taken root in age-oriented or developmental specialties in psychiatry. It is, or should be, as I have indicated, impossible for a geriatric psychiatrist to avoid awareness of the impact of societal forces on the adaptation and maladaptation of older people in any culture or subculture. To a significant extent the psychiatrists interested in adolescence and youth show a higher than average interest in social factors influencing those particular populations (Offer 1969). Analogously, widespread problem areas such as hard drug use (including alcoholism), violence, identity crises, and a host of other related matters are inexplicable without consideration of social variables. Biological and psychological processes, for example, may be the key independent variables to explain a significant number of individual cases of violent behavior, but they cannot adequately explain the high or low incidence of such behavior in particular groups. Biological processes certainly determine major components of behavioral variance at puberty, at menopause (male and female), and in old age. In each case, however, social variables interact with the biological, and the concept of sociobiology is quite relevant to developmental studies of human behavior throughout the life cycle.

All of the above forces, however, were not sufficient to catalyze the social psychiatric confluence of the early 1960s. It is widely recognized that the prime mover came from developments within hospital psychiatry during the 1950s (Stanton and Schwartz 1954; Sabshin 1962). Indeed, in my opinion the most significant development of American psychiatry in the 1950s was the *interaction of social reorganization within our psychiatric hospitals and the effects of the newer medications.* I emphasize the interaction of these two developments which in themselves constitute another excellent example of sociobiological transactions. Hospital psychiatry of the 1950s moved toward an interesting blend of pragmatic service and theory-building. Milieu therapy evolved as a significant acknowledgment that social structure, role function, group processes, and the relationship between the hospital and its surround were salient variables affecting the behavior of patients *and* staff. The pragmatism led to a variety of practices based at the beginning primarily on faith, hope, and enthusiasm: patient participation in the decision-making process should be wide; patient government is a good thing because it is more democratic; staff hierarchy produces tension and a team approach is needed, although it was not always clear whether one was proposing a volleyball team or a football team; * hospitals should no longer be isolated from the community, and the principle of increased permeability across closed doors was honored in an almost compulsive ritual.

Significantly, however, the hospital social psychiatry of the 1950s demonstrated a steady increase in research during the course of the decade. Sociologists, psychologists, and anthropologists joined with their social psychiatric colleagues to make the mental hospital a viable field for scientific investigation. By 1960 the research yield from those studies had an impact upon hospital practice and, in some cases, contributed to the knowledge of organizational systems in general. *Social psychiatry had achieved considerable momentum in 1960 with hospital psychiatry leading the way.* In a 1961 paper I commented: "A frequency distribution of the use of the words, 'social psychiatry,' in our literature would indicate a geometric rise in utilization over the past ten years. *I believe ten years from now the movement will be expanded and institutionalized significantly.* Newer organizational forms will develop, including research centers and training programs" (Sabshin 1962). Twelve years after that predictive statement I can state most definitely that my prediction was wrong. In fact, the words, *social psychiatry* are less frequently used now than in 1961 and the institutionalization has barely occurred in the United States.

What came, of course, was the rapid shift in direction toward community psychiatry, in itself partially a sequel of the earlier developments in hospital psychiatry. Quite correctly, the opening of lines between the outside world and the psychiatric hospitals shifted the locus of care closer to the patient's residence. Legislation supporting community mental health programs catalyzed this trend and resulted in vigorous efforts to seek alternatives to hos-

* Football teams have much greater role differentiation and a vertical chain of command.

pitalization. To some extent a new stigma against the psychiatric hospital began to be manifested in a view which equated the need to hospitalize a patient with failure in community care. In such a context, bright young psychiatrists began to opt for work where the action was—in the community; hospital psychiatry, with a few notable exceptions, gradually withered. In my judgment, this move toward the community was correct from a moral as well as from a pragmatic basis. It was also correct in terms of scientific potential and research possibilities. Unfortunately, the world of community mental health and the changing delivery systems associated with it became so embroiled in the social conflicts of the 1960s that science had a low priority. In a 1965 paper (Sabshin 1968) I predicted that such low priority would become an Achilles' heel of significance when the days of stern accountability and evaluation arrived. This gloomy prediction has proven partially correct; we are now experiencing considerable difficulty in justifying continuation of community mental health programs. Social psychiatry also suffered a setback as a by-product of these developments. Rampant pragmatism and the emphasis on action and applications inhibited scholarly investigations, and this has been a serious loss, in my judgment. Furthermore, critics of community mental health have particularly emphasized the sociopolitical nature of the field and have denigrated its scientific or intellectual possibilities.

Social Psychiatric Research

My concern with lost momentum and lost opportunities in social psychiatric research accounts in part for my collaboration with Brodie (1973) in conducting an overview of recent trends in psychiatric research. One paper on this subject appeared as the lead article in the December issue of the *American Journal of Psychiatry*. I wish to summarize a few salient points.

In this paper we analyzed selected publications during the decade 1963–72. Our key methodological decision involved the selection of publications considered potentially valid indicators of a decade's research trends. We ultimately decided to select the *Archives of General Psychiatry* and the *American Journal of Psychiatry* because they have general rather than specialized psychiatric content and by far the widest circulation of the psychiatric journals. Arbitrary exclusion of other published material may, of course, produce a number of significant artifacts. The omission of books, monographs, and other journals within the field of psychiatry and outside of it may skew the results and is thus a basis for limiting our conclusions. During the decade 1963–72, 4,103 papers were published in the *Archives of General Psychiatry* and the *American Journal of Psychiatry;* each was reviewed and classified as either research or nonresearch. Our study then focused on the 1,885 (46 percent) research articles as well as on hypothesis-testing presentations.

We attempted to categorize the research papers further in three major subdivisions. Since little previous effort has been made to categorize research publications, the variables selected in this paper were necessarily tentative and preliminary. The 1885 research papers were sorted by year, *first* of all as to whether the primary thrust (in most cases, the independent variable of the investigation) of the study involved biological, psychological, or social variables. Since most etiological theories in psychiatry can be sorted into one of these three perspectives, it appeared logical to utilize this classification as a starting point. Furthermore, similar terminology has proven useful in categorizing psychiatric treatments (e.g., somatotherapeutic, psychotherapeutic, sociotherapeutic) (Strauss et al. 1964).

After the biological, psychological, and social variables had been chosen at least in part because of their pertinence to etiology and treatment, a *second* decision was made concerning whether the papers were primarily reporting studies on etiology or treatments. It became necessary to add a third category which we called "mechanisms," since a large part of psychiatric research falls somewhere between etiology and treatment. To some extent our "mechanism" variable is an ambiguous term covering a wide range of data, and we presume that increasing clarity in our understanding of psychiatric disorders will lead to a more precise definition of these intervening variables.

Forty-one percent of the research articles published in the *Archives of General Psychiatry* and the *American Journal of Psychiatry* over the decade focused on biological studies, 35 percent on psychological studies, and 24 percent on social studies. Only 6 percent of the research papers in this period focused primarily on etiology; 30 percent focused on treatment and 64 percent on mechanisms.

To return to my specific topic today—one of the striking findings of this survey involves the paucity of publications related to social causation of psychiatric illness. Only 10 papers on this subject were published! Social psychiatric concepts had included several significant etiological formulations during the 1950s, and by the beginning of the 1960s it appeared that we were on the verge of developing new constructs regarding social variables as specific determinants of psychopathology. Quite clearly, these new constructs have not emerged between 1963 and 1972, and this void may represent a significant commentary on the past decade. One of the most important questions about this issue relates to the emphasis on pragmatic programs during the 1960s as contrasted to theory-building. Papers on "Delivery of Mental Health" represented a large component of the nonresearch published papers. It is conceivable that these efforts siphoned off potential research on social etiology. There may be other explanations, but we must still face the possibility that social factors may prove to be secondary or tertiary variables rather than primary etiological determinants in psychiatric syndromes. The data from the past decade appear to continue to support the hypothesis that social factors may influence all psychiatric phenomena from a mild to moderate degree, but there is no solid evidence of a stronger predictive or causative role of social variables.

One hundred twenty-two research papers on social *treatment* modalities have been published in the *American Journal of Psychiatry* and the *Archives of General Psychiatry* during the past decade. The frequency of such papers seems slightly higher toward the latter part of the 10-year period, with 1971 the peak year.

The 1963 and 1964 papers were significantly concerned with hospital psychiatry; these publications continued the interest in the psychiatric hospital as a social system, a dominant motif during the 1950s (Stanton and Schwartz 1954; Caudill 1958), as indicated. It should be noted, however, that several of the 1963 papers involved general hospital psychiatry. These reflect a rapid increase in the use of this type of hospital as a therapeutic setting (Errera et al. 1963; Smith and McKerracher 1964).

By the latter part of the decade surveyed in this report, the focus on milieu therapy had receded significantly; in fact, papers on hospital psychiatry declined in number and changed in theme. Consideration of the interface between the hospital and the community replaced the more specific investigation of the hospital's social structure, and alternatives to hospitalization emerged as a common subject.

Other themes more common in published research in the latter part of the decade than in the earlier period included: social system variables as they impinged upon drug abuse; newer types of group approaches; and special types of urban psychiatric problems (Stubblebine and Decker 1971). In the nonresearch papers these themes and others related to the delivery of mental health services were even more common, reflecting a significant interest in the search for a more equitable distribution of psychiatric services.

Research support for *primary prevention* remains quite sparse. We probably will never duplicate the contribution of the treatment of neurosyphilis with psychosis and paresis made by the introduction of penicillin, but we should be further along on primary prevention of psychosis with specific high-risk groups.

Another striking finding is the paucity of specific innovations of therapeutic techniques in the community contexts. Most of the energy and the effort involved the creation and survival of clinics; there appeared to be little time or inclination to explore novel therapies.

By almost any criteria the publications on social mechanism represent a heterogeneous group. They vary from transcultural analyses (Brody 1966) to social psychological studies of major political events during the decade. The epidemiology of mental illness continued to receive attention (Leighton et al. 1963; McKegney 1967), as did alcoholism, suicide, accidents, forensic psychiatry, violence (West 1967), and the social readjustment of former patients (Levenstein et al. 1966). Toward the latter part of the decade there were relatively more papers on drug use and abuse (Freedman 1968; Lipp and Beason 1972), racism (Comer 1969; Sabshin et al. 1970; Jones et al. 1970), problems among soldiers and veterans, and student mental health on the college campus (Reifler and Liptzin 1969). Newer concerns with ecology ("ecopsychiatry") had not yet reached the psychiatric journals under our purview, nor had the significant interest in sexism (Bart 1972) been reflected in published research reports in these same journals.

The social mechanism papers when reviewed as a whole did not produce any striking new breakthroughs. Their diverse character and large number appear to indicate a significant attempt to grope with important social psychiatric issues, but the outcome of this massive and complex effort is still to be determined.

Biological research continued its preemptive position during the decade but appears to have diminished toward the latter part of the 10-year period. The number of social papers increased, but most involved "mechanisms" and are heterogeneous and without clear directions. By and large, psychiatric research is still equated with biological research, at least in the minds of influential thinkers. Furthermore, concern is felt in some quarters lest studies of social variables exceed the boundaries of psychiatry, and many colleagues fear that these interests jeopardize the primacy of the medical model. Taken in juxtaposition, a biobehavioral definition of research and a somewhat defensive stand within an *arx medica* have increased the difficulty of recruiting bright young psychiatrists for social psychiatric research.

Nevertheless, I see encouraging trends also. The West Germans have picked up some of the slack (Dörner and Plog 1972), and the British have remained steadier than we have (Bennett 1973). The many papers on social mechanisms imply continued groping, and the large number of nonresearch papers indicates an interest in social and community approaches that is still quite high.

I remain optimistic that we shall be able some day to find a blend of that enlightened humanism which glowed so warmly in the era of moral treatment with the scientific positivism and transactional system approaches of this century. A bicentennial perspective is a superb antidote to overestimation of the *problems* as well as the *solutions* of our current period.

Bibliography

Bart, P.: The myth of a value-free psychotherapy. In *The Sociology of the Future*. Bell, W., and Mau, J. (eds.). New York: The Russell Sage Foundation, 1972, pp. 113–59.

Bennett, D.: Community mental health in Great Britain. *American Journal of Psychiatry* 130:1065–71, 1973.

Bockhoven, J. S.: *Moral Treatment in American Psychiatry*. New York: Springer, 1963.

Brodie, H., Keith, H., and Sabshin, M.: An overview of trends in psychiatric research: 1963–1972. *American Journal of Psychiatry* 130:1309–18, 1973.

Brody, E. B.: Recording cross-culturally useful psychiatric interview data: Experience from Brazil. *American Journal of Psychiatry* 123:446–56, 1966.

Caudill, W. A.: *The Psychiatric Hospital as a Small Society*. Cambridge, Mass.: Harvard University Press, 1958.

Comer, J. P.: White racism: Its root, form, and function. *American Journal of Psychiatry* 126:802–6, 1969.

Dörner, K., and Plog, U.: Sozialpsychiatrie. *Sammlung Luchterhand* 66, June 1972.

Dreikurs, R.: Early experiments in social psychiatry. *International Journal of Social Psychiatry* 7:141–47, 1961.

Errera, P., Wyshak, G., and Jarecki, H.: Psychiatric care in a general hospital emergency room. *Archives of General Psychiatry* 9:105–12, 1963.

Freedman, D. X.: On the use and abuse of LSD. *Archives of General Psychiatry* 18:330–47, 1968.

Holmstrom, R.: On the picture of mental health. *Acta Psychiatrica Scandinavica. Suppl.* 231, 1972.

Jones, B. F., Lightfoot, O. B., Palmer, D., et al. Problems of black psychiatric residents in white training institutions. *American Journal of Psychiatry* 127:798–803, 1970.

Kardiner, A.: *The Individual and His Society*. New York: Columbia University Press, 1939.

——, and Ovesey, L.: *The Mark of Oppression: A Psychosocial Study of the American Negro*. New York: W. W. Norton, 1951.

Kramer, M.: Cross-national study of diagnosis of the mental disorders: Origin of the problem. *American Journal of Psychiatry* 125 (suppl.) :1–11, 1969.

Leighton, D. C., Harding, J. S., Macklin, D. E., et al. Psychiatric findings of the Stirling County Study. *American Journal of Psychiatry* 119:1021–26, 1963.

Levenstein, S., Klein, D. F., and Pollack, M.: Follow-up study of formerly hospitalized voluntary psychiatric patients: The first two years. *American Journal of Psychiatry* 122:1102–9, 1966.

Lipp, M. R., and Benson, S. G.: Physician use of marijuana, alcohol, and tobacco. *American Journal of Psychiatry* 129:612–16, 1972.

McKegney, F. P.: The incidence and characteristics of patients with conversion reactions. I.A general hospital consultation service sample. *American Journal of Psychiatry* 124:542–45, 1967.

Offer, D.: *The Psychological World of the Teen-Ager: A Study of Normal Adolescent Boys*. New York: Basic Books, 1969.

——, and Sabshin, M.: *Normality: Theoretical and Clinical Concepts of Mental Health*. New York: Basic Books, 1966; 2d ed., 1974.

Reifler, C. B., and Liptzin, M. B.: Epidemiological studies of college mental health. *Archives of General Psychiatry* 20:528–40, 1969.

Sabshin, M.: Current perspectives in social psychiatry. Paper presented before the Illinois Psychiatric Society, Chicago, Ill., April 18, 1962.

——: The boundaries of community psychiatry. *The Social Service Review* 40:246–54, 1966a.

——: Theoretical models in community and social psychiatry. In *Community Psychiatry*. Roberts, L. M., Halleck, S. L., and Loeb, M. (eds.). Madison: University of Wisconsin Press, 1966b, pp. 15–30.

——: Toward more rigorous definitions of mental health. In *Comprehensive Mental Health: The Challenge of Evaluation*. Roberts, L. M., Greenfield, N. S., and Miller, M. H. (eds.). Madison: University of Wisconsin Press, 1968.

——, Diesenas, H., and Wilkerson, R.: Dimensions of institutional racism in psychiatry. *American Journal of Psychiatry* 127:787–93, 1970.

Smith, C. M., McKerracher, D. G.: The comprehensive psychiatric unit in the general hospital. *American Journal of Psychiatry* 121:52–57, 1964.

Stanton, A. H., and Schwartz, M. S.: *The Mental Hospital: A Study of Institutional Participation in Psychiatric Illness and Treatment*. New York: Basic Books, 1954.

Strauss, A., Schatzman, L., Bucher, R., Ehrlich, D., and Sabshin, M. *Psychiatric Ideologies and Institutions*. New York: Free Press of Glencoe, 1964.

Stubblebine, J. M., and Decker, J. B.: Are urban mental health centers worth it? *American Journal of Psychiatry* 127:908–12, 1971.

Sullivan, H. S.: Socio-psychiatric research: Its implications for the schizophrenia problem and for mental hygiene. *American Journal of Psychiatry* 10, 1931.

West, L. J.: The psychobiology of racial violence. *Archives of General Psychiatry* 16:645–51, 1967.

Yalom, I. D., et al.: *Encounter Groups and Psychiatry*. Report of the American Psychiatric Association's Task Force on Recent Developments in the Use of Small Groups. Task Force Report no. 1. Washington, D.C.: American Psychiatric Association, April 1970.

9. Implications of Expected Changes in Composition of U.S. Population for the Delivery of Mental Health Services during the Period 1971-85

Morton Kramer, SC.D.

THE subject of this meeting is most relevant to the program of the Biometry Branch of the National Institute of Mental Health. I therefore appreciate very much the opportunity to make these comments.

One of the major objectives of the epidemiological and statistical research that we carry out at NIMH is to provide systematic, uniform historical data on trends in the frequency of occurrence of mental disorders, and the patterns of use of psychiatric services in the United States (Group for the Advancement of Psychiatry 1961; Kramer 1969; Kramer et al. 1955; Kramer and Pollack 1958; Morris 1964; Pollack and Taube 1973; Taube et al. 1973). Such data provide quantitative measures of change in the care of the mentally ill that result from applying available knowledge in order to modify the amount of mental disorder within a population (American Public Health Association 1962). These data may also be used to make projections to estimate future needs for mental health services and the resources needed to deliver these services. For example, how many persons are likely to be in need of psychiatric services, say, in 1985? How many facilities and personnel will we need to provide these services? We are most interested in determining what can be done to reduce the number of persons who acquire one or another kind of mental disorder; to shorten the duration of those disorders which have already occurred; to reduce the amount of disability and distress caused by disorders that are unpreventable and nonterminable. In short, we are concerned about resources needed to apply our knowledge of the prevention and treatment of mental disorders in the most effective, efficient, and economic way possible. These issues are assuming greater and greater importance in furthering community mental health programs, as well as in the development of plans for National Health Insurance, which will include some as yet undetermined package of benefits for the treatment of mental disorders.

In this paper I shall provide a limited number of facts which, I believe, are important for the psychiatric profession to be aware of in developing strategies to deal more effectively with problems to be anticipated in the not-too-distant future. Consideration of such data is also important to tomorrow's panelists in their discussions of the future role and viability of psychiatry.

Change in Patterns of Use of Psychiatric Facilities

Striking changes have taken place in the locus of the delivery of mental health services—from the "isolated and neglected wards of the State hospitals to the newly created but not always adequate facilities in the community" (Eisenberg 1973). These changes are illustrated in tables 1 and 2, which document trends in the use of psychiatric facilities in the United States since 1955, the year in which the first decrease occurred in the nation's state mental hospital population after more than 100 years of continuous increase. In 1955, these hospitals accounted for 818,832 patient care episodes, or 505 per 100,000 population. This number was about half of the total episodes provided by all the psychiatric facilities operating in the United States at the time. By 1971, the number of patient care episodes provided by state mental hospitals was 745,259, a rate of 363 per 100,000. This number was 18.3 percent of the episodes provided by all facilities then operating. In 1971, eight years after the passage of the Community Mental Health Centers Act, the operating federally funded centers accounted for a higher number of episodes (796,647) than the state mental hospitals (745,259).

Figure 1 shows the changes between 1966 and 1971 in the annual rates of patient care episodes specific for age and type of facility. During this interval the total patient care episodes provided by all of these facilities increased from 2.8 million to 4.0 million, and the corresponding rates from 1,427 to 1,989 per 100,000 population. The increase in rates in the age group 25–44 years was striking—from 2,000 per 100,000 in 1966, to 3,000 per 100,000 in 1971. There was also considerable increase in services provided to children under 18 (from 500 to about 1,100

Table 1. Number and percent of patient care episodes and rate per 100,000 population, by type of psychiatric facility: United States, 1946, 1955, 1963, 1971

Type of psychiatric facility	1946	1955	1963	1971
	No. of patient care episodes			
All facilities	870,560 [a]	1,675,352 [b]	2,235,940 [b]	4,081,796
Mental hospitals	762,108	1,030,418	1,037,286	1,020,022
State and county	587,568	818,832	799,401	745,259
Veterans	91,655	88,355	109,973	176,800
Private	82,888	123,231	127,912	97,963
Psychiatric services of general hospitals	108,452	265,934	349,654	542,642
Outpatient psychiatric clinics	NR	379,000	849,000	1,693,848
Residential treatment centers for emotionally disturbed children	NR	NR	NR	28,637
Community mental health centers	NA	NA	NA	796,647
	%			
All facilities	c	100.0	100.0	100.0
Mental hospitals	c	61.5	46.4	25.0
State and county	c	48.9	35.7	18.3
Veterans	c	5.3	4.9	4.3
Private	c	7.3	5.7	2.4
Psychiatric services of general hospitals	c	15.9	15.6	13.3
Outpatient psychiatric clinics	c	22.6	38.0	41.5
Residential treatment centers for emotionally disturbed children	c	d	d	0.7
Community mental health centers	c	NA	NA	19.5
	Rate per 100,000 population			
All facilities	629.1	1,032.2 [b]	1,197.8 [b]	1,989.1
Mental hospitals	550.7	634.8	555.7	497.1
State and county	424.6	504.5	428.2	363.2
Veterans	66.2	54.4	58.9	86.2
Private	59.9	75.9	68.5	47.7
Psychiatric services of general hospitals	78.4	163.8	187.3	264.4
Outpatient psychiatric clinics	NR	233.5	454.8	825.4
Residential treatment centers for emotionally disturbed children	NR	NR	NR	14.0
Community mental health centers	NA	NA	NA	388.2

SOURCE: Data are from Biometry Branch, OPPE, NIMH, ADAMHA.
NOTE: NR = not reported; NA = not applicable (community mental health centers were not in existence in these years).
[a] Total excludes outpatient psychiatric clinics and residential treatment centers which did not report.
[b] Total excludes residential treatment centers.
[c] Percent distribution not computed due to nonreporting of some types of facilities.
[d] Although data were not reported in these years, percentages were probably less than 1 percent.

Table 2. Percent change in numbers and in rates per 100,000 population of patient care episodes, by type of psychiatric facility: United States, 1946–71

Type of psychiatric facility	1946–55	1955–63	1963–71
	% change in nos.		
All facilities	a	a	a
Mental hospitals	35.2	.7	− 1.7
State and county	39.4	− 2.4	− 6.8
Veterans	− 3.6	24.5	60.8
Private	48.7	3.8	−23.4
Psychiatric services of general hospitals	145.2	31.5	55.2
Outpatient psychiatric clinics	a	124.0	99.5
Residential treatment centers for emotionally disturbed children	a	a	a
Community mental health centers	b	b	b
	% change in rates per 100,000 population		
All facilities	a	a	a
Mental hospitals	15.3	−12.5	−10.5
State and county	18.8	−15.0	−15.2
Veterans	−17.8	8.5	46.3
Private	26.7	− 9.6	−30.4
Psychiatric services of general hospitals	108.9	14.4	41.2
Outpatient psychiatric clinics	a	94.9	81.5
Residential treatment centers for emotionally disturbed children	a	a	a
Community mental health centers	b	b	b

SOURCE: Data are from Biometry Branch, OPPE, NIMH, ADAMHA.
[a] Not computed due to nonreporting for outpatient clinics in 1946 and for residential treatment centers in 1946, 1955, and 1963.
[b] Not computed since community mental health centers were not in existence in 1946, 1955, and 1963.

episodes per 100,000). On the other side of the age spectrum, there was a decrease in services provided to persons 65 years and over—from 1,600 to 1,300 episodes per 100,000.

Figure 2 shows the extraordinary change that has taken place in the role of mental hospitals—state and county, VA and private—in providing services to the aged mentally ill. The nursing home has steadily replaced these facilities as the primary locus for the care of these persons. In 1963, 47 percent of mentally disordered persons 65 years and over, and resident in either a mental hospital or nursing home, were in mental hospitals, and 53 percent in nursing homes. By 1969, the corresponding proportions were 25 percent and 75 percent, respectively.

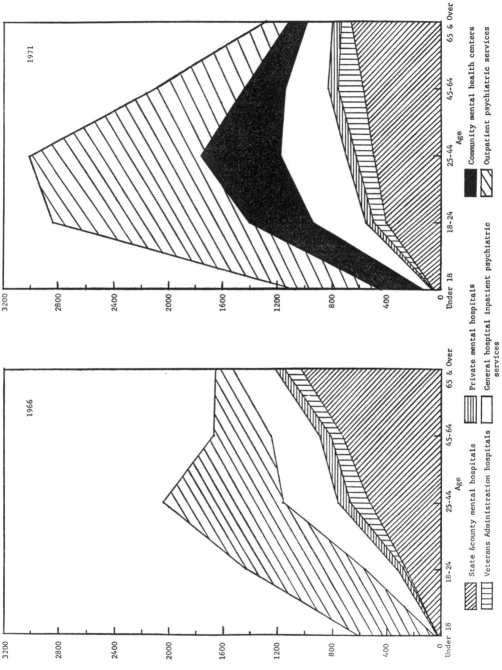

Fig. 1 Number of patient care episodes per 100,000 population in psychiatric facilities by type of facility, by age: United

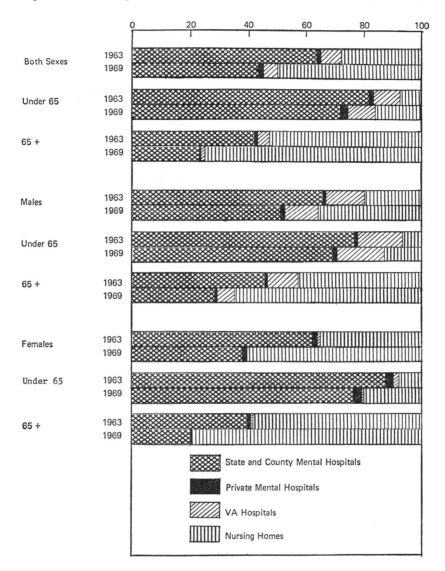

Fig. 2. Percent distribution of patients with mental disorders resident in selected long-term institutions by age and sex: United States, 1963, 1969 (Based on data from Biometry Branch, OPPE, NIMH, ADAMHA)

Patient Care Episodes in 1971
by Sex, Diagnosis, and Type of Facility

Changes have also occurred in the caseload of mental hospitals and other psychiatric facilities in respect to age, sex, and diagnosis. The tables documenting these changes are too numerous to include here.* It is of interest, however, to consider the patterns of use of the various facilities, by sex and diagnosis, during 1971. The details are shown in table 3 and the highlights will be summarized here.

For all facilities combined, schizophrenia was the leading diagnostic category, accounting for 22 percent of all patient care episodes, followed by depressive disorders (15 percent), alcohol disorders (9 percent), organic brain syndromes (5 percent), mental retardation (3 percent), drug disorders (3 percent). The diagnostic distributions varied markedly by sex. There was also considerable variation by type of facility. For example, depressive disorders accounted for only 9 percent of total episodes (both sexes combined) in state and county hospitals, but for a considerably higher proportion of the episodes in private mental hospitals (38 percent), general hospital inpatient psychiatric units (31 percent), and inpatient services of community mental health centers (25 percent). There were also marked differences between patient care episodes in outpatient and inpatient facilities.

Many factors have operated over the years to produce the situation existing in 1971. Indeed, data of the type just discussed can serve as the starting point for studies of such key issues as socioeconomic, attitudinal, and geographical factors that account for differential patterns of use of specific types of facilities by various subgroups of our population; the effectiveness and efficiency of services rendered; methods of payment for services; manpower needs; gaps in services; relationships of psychiatric facilities to one another, as well as to other human-service agencies.

* "Historical Tables on Changes in Patterns of Use of Psychiatric Facilities, 1946–71," available from the Biometry Branch, OPPE, NIMH, ADAMHA, 5600 Fishers Lane, Rockville, Maryland 20852.

Table 3. Number, percent distribution, and rates per 100,000 population of patient care episodes by diagnosis and sex, by type of psychiatric facility: United States, 1971

Sex and diagnosis	All facilities	Inpatient services					Outpatient services	
		State and county mental hospitals	Private mental hospitals	VA hospitals	General hospital psychiatric units (excluding VA)	Community mental health centers	Community mental health centers	Other
				No. of patient care episodes				
Both sexes	4,009,506	745,259	97,963	176,800	542,642	130,088	622,906	1,693,848
Mental retardation	122,609	40,227	302	233	3,495	2,509	23,588	52,255
Organic brain syndrome	216,153	104,015	5,292	18,627	24,573	5,184	12,903	45,559
Schizophrenia	901,119	283,462	22,289	60,045	142,493	28,885	62,934	301,011
Depressive disorders	615,261	65,420	37,422	21,099	165,749	32,018	80,135	213,418
Other psychoses	61,851	7,785	2,568	1,330	11,078	5,049	7,383	26,658
Alcohol disorders	353,020	125,022	8,782	32,456	45,563	15,803	39,483	35,911
Drug disorders	117,069	28,513	2,686	4,455	27,333	5,175	21,612	27,295
All other	1,300,728	74,300	17,051	36,599	109,911	25,542	249,662	787,663
Undiagnosed	321,696	16,515	1,571	1,956	12,447	9,923	125,206	154,078
Males	2,044,576	411,907	39,756	172,433	250,087	59,133	298,985	812,275
Mental retardation	75,790	23,370	156	233	2,762	1,456	13,595	34,218
Organic brain syndromes	118,032	47,595	2,145	18,246	14,201	2,524	7,072	26,249
Schizophrenia	451,824	141,804	8,619	58,158	74,971	12,789	29,426	126,057
Depressive disorders	201,222	22,616	12,009	20,166	45,688	10,142	23,632	66,969
Other psychoses	22,432	2,353	793	1,242	5,539	2,430	2,954	7,121
Alcohol disorders	283,115	101,477	6,239	32,320	33,674	11,690	31,253	66,462
Drug disorders	83,015	20,772	1,549	4,213	18,601	2,743	15,040	20,097
All other	640,113	41,332	7,624	35,899	44,714	10,760	116,669	383,115
Undiagnosed	169,033	10,588	622	1,956	9,937	4,599	59,344	81,987

Source: Data are from Biometry Branch, OPPE, NIMH, ADAMHA.

Table 3 (*cont.*)

Sex and diagnosis	All facilities	Inpatient services					Outpatient services	
		State and county mental hospitals	Private mental hospitals	VA hospitals	General hospital psychiatric units (excluding VA)	Community mental health centers	Community mental health centers	Other
Females	1,964,930	333,352	58,207	4,367	292,555	70,955	323,921	881,573
Mental retardation	46,819	16,857	146	381	733	1,053	9,993	18,037
Organic brain syndromes	98,121	56,420	3,147	1,887	10,372	2,660	5,831	19,310
Schizophrenia	449,295	141,658	13,670	933	67,522	16,096	33,508	174,954
Depressive disorders	414,039	42,804	25,413	88	120,661	21,876	56,503	146,449
Other psychoses	39,419	5,432	1,775	136	5,539	2,619	4,429	19,537
Alcohol disorders	69,905	23,545	2,543	242	11,889	4,113	8,230	19,449
Drug disorders	34,054	7,741	1,137	700	8,732	2,432	6,572	7,198
All other	660,615	32,968	9,427	—	65,197	14,782	132,993	404,548
Undiagnosed	152,663	5,927	949		2,510	5,324	65,862	72,091
% distribution by diagnosis								
Both sexes	100.0	100.0	100.0	100.0	100.0	100.0	100.0	100.0
Mental retardation	3.1	5.4	0.3	0.1	0.6	1.9	3.8	3.1
Organic brain syndromes	5.4	14.0	5.4	10.5	4.5	4.0	2.1	2.7
Schizophrenia	22.5	38.0	22.8	34.0	26.3	22.2	10.1	17.7
Depressive disorders	15.4	8.8	38.2	11.9	30.6	24.6	12.8	12.6
Other psychoses	1.5	1.0	2.6	0.8	2.0	3.9	1.2	1.6
Alcohol disorders	8.8	16.8	9.0	18.4	8.4	12.2	6.3	5.1
Drug disorders	2.9	3.8	2.7	2.5	5.0	4.0	3.5	1.6
All other	32.4	10.0	17.4	20.7	20.3	19.6	40.1	46.5
Undiagnosed	8.0	2.2	1.6	1.1	2.3	7.6	20.1	9.1

Table 3 (cont.)

Sex and diagnosis	All facilities	Inpatient services					Outpatient services	
		State and county mental hospitals	Private mental hospitals	VA hospitals	General hospital psychiatric units (excluding VA)	Community mental health centers	Community mental health centers	Other
Males	100.0	100.0	100.0	100.0	100.0	100.0	100.0	100.0
Mental retardation	3.7	5.7	0.4	0.1	1.1	2.5	4.5	4.2
Organic brain syndromes	5.8	11.6	5.4	10.6	5.7	4.3	2.4	3.2
Schizophrenia	22.1	34.4	21.7	33.7	30.0	21.6	9.8	15.5
Depressive disorders	9.8	5.5	30.2	11.7	18.3	17.1	7.9	8.3
Other psychoses	1.1	0.6	2.0	0.7	2.2	4.1	1.0	0.9
Alcohol disorders	13.8	24.6	15.7	18.8	13.4	19.8	10.5	8.1
Drug disorders	4.1	5.0	3.9	2.5	7.4	4.6	5.0	2.5
All other	31.3	10.0	19.2	20.8	17.9	18.2	39.0	47.2
Undiagnosed	8.3	2.6	1.5	1.1	4.0	7.8	19.9	10.1
Females	100.0	100.0	100.0	100.0	100.0	100.0	100.0	100.0
Mental retardation	2.4	5.1	0.2	—	0.2	1.5	3.1	2.1
Organic brain syndromes	5.0	16.9	5.4	8.7	3.5	3.8	1.8	2.2
Schizophrenia	22.9	42.5	23.5	43.2	23.1	22.7	10.4	19.8
Depressive disorders	21.1	12.8	43.7	21.4	41.0	30.8	17.4	16.6
Other psychoses	2.0	1.6	3.0	2.0	1.9	3.7	1.4	2.2
Alcohol disorders	3.5	7.1	4.4	3.1	4.1	5.8	2.5	2.2
Drug disorders	1.7	2.3	2.0	5.6	3.0	3.4	2.0	0.8
All other	33.6	9.9	16.2	16.0	22.3	20.8	41.1	45.9
Undiagnosed	7.8	1.8	1.6	—	0.9	7.5	20.3	8.2

Table 3 (*cont.*)

Sex and diagnosis	All facilities	Inpatient services					Outpatient services	
		State and county mental hospitals	Private mental hospitals	VA hospitals	General hospital psychiatric units (excluding VA)	Community mental health centers	Community mental health centers	Other
		Rate per 100,000 population						
Both sexes	1953.8	363.2	47.7	86.2	264.4	63.4	303.5	825.4
Mental retardation	59.7	19.6	0.1	0.1	1.7	1.2	11.5	25.5
Organic brain syndromes	105.3	50.7	2.6	9.1	12.0	2.5	6.3	22.2
Schizophrenia	439.1	138.1	10.9	29.3	69.4	14.1	30.7	146.7
Depressive disorders	299.8	31.9	18.2	10.3	80.8	15.6	39.0	104.0
Other psychoses	30.1	3.8	1.3	0.6	5.4	2.5	3.6	13.0
Alcohol disorders	172.0	60.9	4.3	15.8	22.2	7.7	19.2	41.9
Drug disorders	57.0	13.9	1.3	2.2	13.3	2.5	10.5	13.3
All other	633.8	36.2	8.3	17.8	53.6	12.4	121.7	383.8
Undiagnosed	156.8	8.0	0.8	1.0	6.1	4.8	61.0	75.1
Males	2049.2	412.8	39.8	172.8	250.7	59.3	299.7	814.1
Mental retardation	76.0	23.4	0.2	0.2	2.8	1.5	13.6	34.3
Organic brain syndromes	118.3	47.7	2.1	18.3	14.2	2.5	7.1	26.3
Schizophrenia	452.9	142.1	8.6	58.3	75.1	12.8	29.5	126.3
Depressive disorders	201.7	22.7	12.0	20.2	45.8	10.2	23.7	67.1
Other psychoses	22.5	2.4	0.8	1.2	5.6	2.4	3.0	7.1
Alcohol disorders	283.8	101.7	6.3	32.4	33.8	11.7	31.3	66.6
Drug disorders	83.2	20.8	1.6	4.2	18.6	2.7	15.1	20.1
All other	641.6	41.4	7.6	36.0	44.8	10.8	116.9	384.0
Undiagnosed	169.4	10.6	0.6	2.0	10.0	4.6	59.5	82.2

Table 3 (*cont.*)

		Inpatient services					Outpatient services	
Sex and diagnosis	All facilities	State and county mental hospitals	Private mental hospitals	VA hospitals	General hospital psychiatric units (excluding VA)	Community mental health centers	Community mental health centers	Other
Females	1863.5	316.2	55.2	4.1	277.5	67.3	307.2	836.1
Mental retardation	44.4	16.0	0.1	—	0.7	1.0	9.5	17.1
Organic brain syndromes	93.1	53.5	3.0	0.4	9.8	2.5	5.5	18.3
Schizophrenia	426.1	134.3	13.0	1.8	64.0	15.3	31.8	165.9
Depressive disorders	392.7	40.6	24.1	0.9	113.9	20.7	53.6	138.9
Other psychoses	37.4	5.2	1.7	0.1	5.3	2.5	4.2	18.5
Alcohol disorders	66.3	22.3	2.4	0.1	11.3	3.9	6.9	18.4
Drug disorders	32.3	7.3	1.1	0.2	8.3	2.3	6.2	6.8
All other	626.5	31.3	8.9	0.7	61.8	14.0	126.1	383.7
Undiagnosed	144.8	5.6	0.9	—	2.4	5.0	62.5	68.4

Implications of Changes in Size and Composition of
the Population of the United States
for Psychiatric Facilities and Manpower

I should like to use the data on use of psychiatric facilities to illustrate their implications for psychiatry and other mental health professions when viewed against forecasts of the size and composition of the general population of the United States by 1980 and 1985. Table 4 shows that by 1985 the population of the United States will have increased to about 241.7 million people, about 19 percent more than in 1970. The increase for whites will be 18 percent (from 177.7 to 209.4 million), and for nonwhites, 27 percent (from 25.5 to 32.3 million). Nonwhites are expected to constitute about 13 percent of the population in 1985. Large relative increases are expected in each age group for the nonwhite population, ranging from a 79 percent increase in the age group 25–34 years, to 9 percent in the age group 45–64. These increases are considerably in excess of those in the white population, which range from 61 percent in the age group 25–34, to 2 percent in the age group 45–64. Of particular importance are the large increases anticipated in age groups that past experience has shown to have consistently high admission rates to psychiatric facilities.

The expected percent changes in the numbers of persons in the various age groups have many implications for the planning of psychiatric services, particularly those provided by state and county mental hospitals, private hospitals with psychiatric services, VA hospitals, outpatient psychiatric services and community mental health centers. For example, if we merely maintained the 1970 level of services to the population through 1985 for persons in the age group 25–34, the *number of episodes* that would be experienced by all the persons in that age group would be *63 percent greater* than the corresponding number in 1970. The increase for the white population would be 61 percent, and for nonwhites, 79 percent.

Table 5 illustrates the extent to which the aforelisted facilities would be meeting the needs of the population for services under varying assumptions of need. Under any estimate of need—2 percent, 10 percent, and 20 percent—the extent of unmet need is considerable, and this will continue to be the case.

Table 4. U.S. populations, actual 1970 and estimated 1985, and numerical and percent change, 1970–85, by age and color

Age	1970			1985		
	Total	White	Nonwhite	Total	White	Nonwhite
	Population (in 000s)					
Total	203,212	177,749	25,463	241,731	209,427	32,304
Under 18	69,644	59,062	10,582	73,307	61,363	11,944
18–24	23,697	20,592	3,105	28,423	23,975	4,448
25–34	24,907	21,779	3,128	40,699	35,109	5,590
35–44	23,089	20,328	2,761	31,384	27,657	3,727
45–64	41,810	37,658	4,152	42,941	38,398	4,543
65 and over	20,066	18,330	1,736	24,977	22,925	2,052
	Change in no. of persons (in 000s), 1970–85			% change in number of persons, 1970–85		
Total	38,519	31,678	6,841	19.0	17.8	26.9
Under 18	3,663	2,301	1,362	5.3	3.9	12.9
18–24	4,726	3,383	1,343	19.9	16.4	43.3
25–34	15,792	13,330	2,462	63.4	61.2	78.7
35–44	8,295	7,329	966	35.9	36.1	35.0
45–64	1,131	740	391	2.7	2.0	9.4
65 and over	4,911	4,595	316	24.5	25.1	18.2

Sources: U.S. Bureau of the Census, Census of Population, 1970. General Population Characteristics PC(1)-B1, table 52; U.S. Bureau of the Census, Current Population Reports, Series P-25, no. 388, tables 2, 6 (Series D Projection).

Table 5. Extent to which needs for psychiatric services would be met in relation to various assumptions of need, assuming 1971 use rates only, by age: United States, 1975, 1980

Age	Estimated gen. pop. (in 000s) (1)	Estimated pt. care episodes (2)	Estimated no. persons recv'g care (3)	Estimated number of persons needing care, assuming:			Number in need not receiving care, assuming:			% unmet need, assuming:		
				2% in need (4)	10% in need (5)	20% in need (6)	2% in need (7)	10% in need (8)	20% in need (9)	2% in need (10)	10% in need (11)	20% in need (12)
1975												
Total	215,324	4,237,576	3,390,061	4,306,480	21,532,400	43,064,800	1,060,510	18,142,339	39,674,739	24.6	84.3	92.1
Under 18	68,109	809,377	647,502	1,362,180	6,810,900	13,621,800	714,678	6,163,398	12,974,298	52.5	90.5	95.2
18-24	27,780	716,150	572,920	555,600	2,778,000	5,556,000	0	2,205,080	4,983,080	0.0	79.4	89.7
25-44	53,835	1,504,340	1,203,471	1,076,700	5,383,500	10,767,000	0	4,180,029	9,563,529	0.0	77.6	88.8
45-64	43,430	932,267	745,814	868,600	4,343,000	8,686,000	122,786	3,597,186	7,940,186	14.1	82.8	91.4
65 and over	24,170	275,442	220,354	443,400	2,217,000	4,434,000	223,046	1,996,646	4,213,646	50.3	90.1	95.0
1980												
Total	228,676	4,500,344	3,600,275	4,573,520	22,867,600	45,735,200	1,030,028	19,267,325	42,134,925	22.5	84.3	92.1
Under 18	69,646	859,566	687,653	1,392,920	6,964,600	13,929,200	705,267	6,276,947	13,241,547	50.6	90.1	95.1
18-24	29,156	760,558	608,446	583,120	2,915,600	5,831,200	0	2,307,154	5,222,754	0.0	79.1	89.6
25-44	62,332	1,597,622	1,278,097	1,246,640	6,233,200	12,466,400	0	4,955,103	11,188,303	0.0	79.5	89.7
45-64	43,489	990,076	792,061	869,780	4,348,900	8,697,800	77,719	3,556,839	7,905,739	8.9	81.8	90.9
65 and over	24,953	292,522	234,018	481,060	2,405,300	4,810,600	247,042	2,171,282	4,576,582	51.4	90.3	95.1

SOURCE: Data for Col. 1 from U.S. Bureau of the Census, Current Population Reports, Series P-25, no. 493 (Series D projection).

Derivation of cols. 2 to 12: Col. 2: Total patient care episodes obtained by applying 1971 patient care episode rate per 100,000 population (1,968 per 100,000) to the projected 1975 and 1980 total U.S. population. Age distribution of patient care episodes obtained by applying 1971 percentage distribution of patient care episodes by age to the 1975 and 1980 estimated total patient care episodes. Col. 3: Represents a conversion of patient care episodes into number of persons accounting for these episodes by multiplying patient care episodes by a factor of 80. This factor was derived from findings of the Maryland Psychiatric Case Register that every person in that register had an average of 1.2 episodes of care per year. Col. 4: Col. 1 X .02. Col. 5: Col. 1 X .10. Col. 6: Col. 1 X .20. Col. 7: Col. 4 − Col. 3. For this column negative values were assumed to be zero, i.e., the need for services would be met. Also the total is the sum of the parts. Col. 8: Col. 5 − Col. 3. Col. 9: Col. 6 − Col. 3. Col. 10: Col. 7 ÷ Col. 4. Col. 11: Col. 8 ÷ Col. 5. Col. 12: Col. 9 ÷ Col. 6.

Table 6 shows the implications of the expected population changes for personnel providing varying levels of services to persons in need. For example, if 10 percent of the population are in need of psychiatric services, then, to provide *six hours per patient per year* of the services of a clinical psychiatrist would require 86,000 psychiatrists in 1975; 91,000 in 1980; and 96,687 in 1985.

The number of professionals needed to provide the various levels of care specified in Table 6 exceeds the expected supply by a considerable amount. This may be illustrated by considering the number of psychiatrists (one or more years of psychiatric training); psychologists (M.A. or Ph.D. with training in mental health field), social workers (M.A. with training in mental health field), and nurses (some training in psychiatric nursing) required to provide *six hours per patient per year per discipline,* assuming a 10-percent level of need for care, as compared to the projected manpower pools for each discipline, in 1975 and 1980:

Discipline	1975		1980	
	Required	Expected *	Required	Expected *
Psychiatry	86,235	30,300	91,004	38,700
Psychology	86,235	30,000	91,004	44,800
Social work	86,235	25,400	91,004	36,600
Nursing	86,235	35,900	91,004	51,300

*Source: Division of Manpower and Training Programs, NIMH.

These computations underscore the sizable increases that may be expected, merely as a result of population increases, in the number of persons needing mental health services, and in the manpower required to deliver these services. I might add that the population forecasts are equally significant for the planning of resources to meet demands for medical care, and for social, welfare, legal, correctional, and other human services, that the expected increases are likely to make.

These computations also emphasize a need for research. If administrators who are planning services are serious about obtaining reliable estimates of need in order to plan programs, to use existing manpower most effectively, to train additional manpower to meet the need, then it is essential that they give a high priority to the design and implementation of the research required to do this. If they are not interested, then estimates of this type or others

Table 6. Estimated number of psychiatrists, psychologists, social workers, and nurses needed to care for all persons in need of psychiatric care assuming various levels of need for care and various amounts of time spent per patient per year: United States 1971, 1975, 1980

Professional discipline and assumed hours per patient per year	Level of need for care, assuming:								
	1971			1975			1980		
	2% in need	10% in need	20% in need	2% in need	10% in need	20% in need	2% in need	10% in need	20% in need
No. of persons in need of care	4,085,080	20,425,400	40,850,800	4,306,480	21,532,400	43,064,800	4,573,520	22,867,600	45,735,200
Clinical psychiatrists									
3 hrs./yr./pt.	8,170	40,851	81,702	8,613	43,065	86,130	9,147	45,735	91,470
6 hrs./yr./pt.	16,340	81,702	163,403	17,226	86,130	172,259	18,294	91,470	182,941
10 hrs./yr./pt.	27,234	136,169	272,339	28,710	143,549	287,099	30,490	152,451	304,901
Psychologists									
3 hrs./yr./pt.	8,170	40,851	81,702	8,613	43,065	86,130	9,147	45,735	91,470
6 hrs./yr./pt.	16,340	81,702	163,403	17,226	86,130	172,259	18,294	91,470	182,941
10 hrs./yr./pt.	27,234	136,169	272,339	28,710	143,549	287,099	30,490	152,451	304,901
Social workers									
6 hrs./yr./pt.	16,340	81,702	163,403	17,226	86,130	172,259	18,294	91,470	182,941
12 hrs./yr./pt.	32,680	163,403	326,806	34,452	172,260	344,518	36,588	182,940	365,882
20 hrs./yr./pt.	54,468	272,339	544,677	57,420	287,099	574,198	60,980	304,901	609,802
Nurses									
6 hrs./yr./pt.	16,340	81,702	163,403	17,226	86,130	172,259	18,294	91,470	182,941
10 hrs./yr./pt.	27,234	136,169	272,339	28,710	143,549	287,099	30,490	152,451	304,901

SOURCE: Number of persons in need of care based on U.S. Bureau of the Census estimated July 1, 1971, civilian resident population (Current Population Reports, Series P-25, no. 490), and U.S. Bureau of the Census, Current Population Reports, Series P-25, no. 493 (Series D projection).

NOTE: It was assumed that each profession would work 50 weeks during the year on an average of 30 hours per week or a total of 1,500 hours per year.

with more elaborate statistical techniques applied to the same inadequate basic data will have to suffice.

In conclusion, the data presented in this paper emphasize the important tasks that face psychiatrists and members of related professions in developing strategies to meet the anticipated increase in needs for mental health services, in terms of facilities, personnel, program content, and financing mechanisms. It is important for directors of federal, state, and local mental health center programs, as well as psychiatrists and other mental health professionals in private practice, to insure that currently available knowledge about the prevention and treatment of mental disorders, and any new knowledge that may be on the horizon, will be applied as effectively, efficiently, and economically as possible during the next decade, and made accessible to all segments of our population equally. By so doing, we will do much to prevent and minimize the disability caused by the mental disorders.

Bibliography

American Public Health Association, Program Area Committee on Mental Health: *Mental Disorder: A Guide to Control Methods.* New York: American Public Health Association, 1962.

Eisenberg, L.: Psychiatric intervention. *Scientific American* 2:116, 1973.

Group for the Advancement of Psychiatry, Committee on Preventive Psychiatry: *Problems of Estimating Changes in Frequency of Mental Disorders.* New York: Group for the Advancement of Psychiatry, 1961.

Kramer, M.: Statistics of mental disorders in the United States: Current status, some urgent needs and suggested solutions (with discussion). *Journal of the Royal Statistical Society* 132:353–407, 1969.

Kramer, M., Goldstein, H., Israel, R. H., and Johnson, N. A.: *An Historical Study of the Disposition of First Admissions to a State Mental Hospital: The Experience of the Warren State Hospital during the Period 1916–1950.* Public Health Monograph no. 32, PHS Publication no. 445. Washington, D.C.: U.S. Government Printing Office, 1955.

Kramer, M., and Pollack, E. S.: Problems in the interpretation of trends in the population movement of the public mental hospitals. *Journal of the American Public Health Association* 48:1003–19, 1958.

Morris, J. N.: *Uses of Epidemiology.* 2d ed. Baltimore: Williams & Wilkins, 1964.

Pollack, E. S., and Taube, C. A.: Trends and projections in state hospital use. Paper presented at the Symposium on the Future Role of the State Hospital, Division of Community Psychiatry, State University of New York at Buffalo, Buffalo, N.Y., 1973.

Taube, C. A., et al.: *Statistical Notes.* Rockville, Md.: Biometry Branch, National Institute of Mental Health, 1969–73.

Discussion

DR. MATHIS: We will now begin the panel discussion on future therapeutic perspectives. It gives us all an opportunity to be as wrong as Dr. Sabshin said he was ten years ago. Certainly we cannot do a double-blind on the future, can we?

I should like to make this program informal. I think it would be good if anyone wishing to interrupt or to ask a question or make a comment at any time felt it appropriate to do so. Perhaps we could start by asking if any panel members wish to make a further verifying statement or to get into future items. Dr. Sabshin says he would rather hear from the audience. We have already had one question from the audience: during the break we were asked for a comment from Dr. Kety on the recently reported use of massive doses of the beta-adrenergic blockers.

DR. KETY: This rather surprising report caused some confusion in people's minds because propranalol is not normally thought to pass the blood-brain barrier to any great extent, and it was not easy to see how it could achieve the results in acute psychotic episodes that were claimed. The use of propranalol in massive doses in the treatment of acute psychotic episodes was replicated, after the earlier report, in one study by John Cole, and the results were much less impressive. In fact, I believe it was not possible to confirm the efficacy of this agent. I think it may very well alleviate some of the symptoms in acute psychosis, but if so it probably does so by blocking the peripheral sympathetic activation which exerts a feedback in a vicious circle, so that the pounding of the heart and other peripheral manifestations may be continually feeding into and exacerbating the central symptoms. But I doubt that we will find in future studies that propranalol is getting at any central aspects of the problem.

DR. ROMANO: May I ask Dr. Sabshin whether he has any constructive suggestions as to how we could avoid the present dilemma in the community health movement, that of catapulting chronic hospitalized patients with little or no social competence into communities in which no resources have been prepared for their reception?

DR. SABSHIN: Let me say, Dr. Romano, that there are other people in this audience more competent to take this up than I am, most notably Dr. Visotsky, Dr. Allerton, and other commissioners—Dr. Visotsky being an ex-commissioner. Some of the events I have described are certainly involved in the issue of moving people out of the hospital too rapidly. Clearly we thought well of custodialism and the long-term hospital stay for so long that it was inevitable that when hospitalization began to seem something necessarily negative we not only admitted to failure when a patient needed hospitalization, but attempted to turn people out of the hospital in a highly pragmatic, ultimately inefficient, and often nonhumanitarian way.

In many states, and particularly in my own, Illinois—and I think Dr. Vistosky and Dr. Grinker would be good people to comment on this—there was an effort to evacuate geriatric patients from hospitals to neighborhoods because the hospitals had become veritable warehouses for the custodial care of geriatric patients. This was attempted in Chicago, where some people, including those I have mentioned, fought against this move because they realized that the resources for such people in the community were inadequate. Their views were countered by a variety of political necessities and the strength of the opposition. Now we begin to hear communities protesting on the basis of very practical reasons, such as the impact on real estate values and the objections of those living next door to patients who had been inadequately prepared to leave the hospital. This situation is a return to some of the problems of the mid-19th century. I am not sure what we can do except to acknowledge this problem and to maximize our influence in trying to bring about a sensible rate of discharge and to develop better resources in the community, where their paucity is still a major problem.

DR. KOLB: I suggest that the problem derives from a number of sources. One of these sources may be, in fact, the extraordinary difference between those who address themselves to the psychology of the individual and those who address themselves to the problems of society at large. When one deals with the problem of the individual patient one is interested in effecting certain changes, one being improvement in his subjective state. I have felt that those who are devising our new techniques or quantifying change have, because of the very difficulty of assessing this kind of change, dedicated themselves to describing the capacity of the individual to perform in one or another socially acceptable way; but they have not focused on what those of you who work with the individual patient are so concerned about—how he feels.

Now the moving of patients into communities where there is inadequate support for them came about, I think, because of a tremendously enthusiastic social attitude that the community was the best place for the patient to be. I fail to recall a single study in which those interested in community and social psychiatry asked a patient whether he wanted to be in the so-called community. For instance, in New York City the move of a patient from a nursing institution in the suburbs to an SRO in central New York—on Broadway, where patients were exposed to violent attacks from other people—became the subject of protest from many families of patients, and others. Studies on how the patient feels about such changes are needed; really, this, too, is a part of social psychiatry. We need to get subjective values into perspective with social values before being pushed ahead by our enthusiasm to demonstrate that we can ship people from one dip of the mental health system into what is in a sense another dip—the community. Furthermore, many communities are quite unprepared, as Dr. Sabshin has said. As a matter of fact, the most accepting communities some of the social scientists have found are those with a middle-class, educated population. Those least prepared to take such patients are the deprived communities already overcrowded with people, many of whom are themselves under considerable stress. One expects to get social protest when returning patients to these communities. We have failed to study how the communities feel about receiving discharged patients, and social studies fail to take into account the feelings of the individual who is moved.

DR. KETY: I think it may be of interest, partly in response to Dr. Romano's question, too, to mention some of the things I learned about Chinese psychiatry on a visit to China in June of this year.

For the first week of my visit it was extremely difficult to find any acknowledgment that mental illness existed in China. I recall that when we met with the medical staff of a large commune of 80,000 outside Canton, I asked about the incidence of acute psychotic episodes there. I was told, "Well, we don't keep records, but it is extremely rare; we don't remember a case of psychosis." (Dr. Kramer's data make very clear the tremendous incidence of psychiatric episodes per 100,000 in America.) We consistently failed to make any contact with psychiatrists, and no psychiatrists were present in the groups of people who greeted us. At one point I felt so desperate about this that when it was my turn to make a toast at a banquet in Peking I toasted "the psychiatrists of China, wherever they may be."

We had a meeting with the minister of health, who turned out to be an extremely enlightened, intelligent, and altogether remarkable man. After he gave us a very modest account of the problems which China faces in public health, the moderate success that they have had, and the areas where they have not as yet made any great impact, we were given the opportunity to ask questions. I indicated that from the little I knew about psychiatry in China, China had eliminated mental illness as a problem, and that if this were the case it would be a much more remarkable achievement than acupuncture anesthesia. I explained that this possibility was the reason why American psychiatrists are so much interested in visiting China and learning more about Chinese psychiatry. I said that when I returned home I was sure my colleagues in America would be very much interested in what I had learned. I asked what he would suggest that I tell them. Should I discourage them from trying to make contact with psychiatrists in China or should I encourage them? Or did he think this a poor time to do the latter? Then he came forward with a very enlightened and sensible statement to the effect that China indeed does have psychiatric problems which are treated, not behind bars, but in open hospitals with milieu therapy, group therapy, and with heavy reliance on some of the modern drugs. He said that they have a great deal to learn about these, and that American friends are welcome to visit at any time, and so forth.

From that moment on everything opened up. I met the senior psychiatrists in China, the professor of psychiatry at Peking, and the professor at Shanghai, and I visited the psychiatric institutions. Now, interestingly enough, in Shanghai, which has a population at least as large as that of New York, psychiatric hospital beds number 2,000—about one-fifth the number of those in New York. I asked the senior psychiatrist to account for this. Schizophrenia is the major mental illness treated in hospitals, and I asked whether schizophrenia is less common in China than in the West. He replied, "No, we think the incidence is the same. But our communities accept the patients more readily and we treat them there. We rely heavily on outpatient services and on phenothiazine drugs, but we do a lot of education of the patient's family and his coworkers so that our patients can be quickly released from the hospital and be accepted by the community."

Of course, as we are learning in Denmark, the prevalence of schizophrenia in rural populations is much lower than in urban populations, and again the difference is probably a reflection of the community's ability to accept or tolerate this kind of deviation. I don't know how the Chinese have succeeded in achieving this remarkable degree of tolerance for mental illness in the community, but I think it may very well be that we could find out.

DR. MATHIS: Dr. Sabshin offered something of a challenge to Drs. Grinker, Visotsky, and Allerton to contribute their thoughts on this subject. May we have some comment from them?

DR. GRINKER: We passed through a very bleak period in Illinois when a lay person was appointed as an interim acting director of the Department of Mental Health. I think there were two reasons why he decided to empty the state hospitals of geriatric patients; first, to make better statistics regarding the populations in the hospitals; and, second, to save money. We of the Psychiatric Council were shocked, and extracted from him a promise that the patients would be prepared over a period of some weeks or months, that there would be inspection of the various community homes to which patients would be discharged, and that continuous care would be provided by mental hospital personnel, who, with fewer patients in the institutions, would then have time to work in the community. Not one of these promises was kept. The patients were summarily discharged to the worst possible area in Chicago, the uptown area, which is populated by poverty-stricken minority groups. As a result these former patients are much worse off than they were in the hospitals, and the death rate is extremely high. And younger people in the community tend to be violent.

I think that the current director is changing things, but—to add emphasis to what Dr. Romano said—unless you maintain the care and supervision of these patients out in the community, discharge from the state hospitals does nothing for them, and fails even to save money for the state. In the context in which Dr. Kety spoke, when the state has a contract with the private psychiatric hospitals for a maximum of 20 days of hospitalization (which means crisis therapy), we found that we were able to discharge about 95 percent of these people back to their communities and their families and their work. The fact is that these poor people are returning to communities that have a high tolerance of deviance, as in the ghettos. Such tolerance of deviance is not found in the middle- and upper-class communities where any anxiety or depression is considered a call for help. The lower socioeconomic group takes back its members with much greater tolerance, and I think that is why the discharge rate is so high.

DR. ARCANGELO D'AMORE: I am Dr. D'Amore from Washington. I don't want to slight Dr. Kolb or Dr. Kety, but I would like to focus on what Dr. Sabshin and Dr. Kramer brought up in terms of a group commonly referred to as the white ethnics—Hungarian Americans, Italian Americans, and so on. I made an amateur statistical study on my 25 years of private practice in Washington, and found that 70 out of 670 private patients I had seen were Italian Americans who came to see me because of my ability to speak Italian. I compared that group with the rest of my practice and found that I had a striking number of elderly patients. I found also that only within the last decade were Italian Americans coming to me for intensive psychotherapy or psychoanalysis, and that in the early years after World War II they wanted some psychosomatic approach, some immediate tranquilization, something immediately available.

Now this group of white ethnics is no longer considered the minority group; they cannot get special funds from the government since public policy does not define them as a minority group. Also, white ethnics have a lot of fierce pride. You will find that they do not want anything resembling a handout or anything that implies that they are weak. They are subjected to the pressure of being considered un-American if they want to perpetuate their ethnic neighborhood, and I have discovered that the typical patient is someone who speaks poor English and prefers to speak Italian, is about 65 years old, lives in a changing neighborhood, and has become depressed and lonely. When you raise the issue of their access to their church and their priest you hear that it is quite a distance on public transportation and they do not get there any more. And there is no support in the neighborhood. They do not qualify for many of the supportive services available to some deprived groups, and so this white ethnic population is in great difficulty.

I would like to hear about this problem from Dr. Sabshin and the others because I find that in the study done in New Haven in 1950, among the more than 600 psychiatric patients in the hospital at that time there was not a single Irish Catholic in individual psychotherapy. There are many problems involved in being able to take advantage of the mental health resources that are available, and others in relation to language barriers and in relation to the support that can be expected from changing neighborhood and family patterns. These tend to give me at least the impression that public policy tends to increase the incidence of mental illness in this group.

Dr. Sabshin: I think this comment is appropriate from a number of angles. I would like to call to your attention studies of the distribution of mental health personnel within large urban complexes. For example, one made in Chicago by Royce and Levy shows that the number of mental health personnel available for white ethnic communities is strikingly low. And it is an interesting point that the distribution in the mental health field of the white ethnics you describe is proportionately much lower than in the population. I think that is an articulation of those two phenomena. These white ethnic areas also report low rates of hospitalization, whatever that means. I would presume that this will change in time because of the spread and diversification in the mental health field. Attitudinal studies in such communities have indicated that such communities are somewhat slower to accept mental health concepts than others are. They have not accepted them, at least, in Chicago. I believe that, too, is changing, and that greater usage will be noted in this part of the city over the next 10 or 15 years. Your comments about your own experiences are an indication of a move in that direction.

The whole issue of hospital prevalence rates raises interesting questions, including what Dr. Kety has said. I should be delighted to see figures from China. I think this is the first time we have heard this news from China, and it is quite impressive. This stage is historically somewhat different for China than for Russia, which, during the period of post–World War I revolution and for several decades thereafter, had a strong need to deny that psychiatric illness was really a problem. Russians needed to believe that they had wiped out a large number of psychiatric problems. It has been only in the last decade that they have to any significant degree acknowledged the extent of their psychiatric problems. I would be wary, of course, as Dr. Kety assumed we all would be, that the prevalence rates in China are more than just a reflection of their agricultural, rural-urban society. The kinds of things he reports are also reported from Burma and, I presume, from Nepal, which has one psychiatrist, who happens to be the editor of that country's medical journal. If you look at the rates there you will see that hospital prevalence rates give you only a very small part of the story, but it is interesting that the Chinese—at least through Dr. Kety's intervention—have opened up to that extent.

Dr. Daniel Blain: The fact that we are here celebrating the anniversary of a historically interesting mental hospital makes it appropriate to say another word about this matter of patients leaving the hospital and getting out into the community. I suggest that this is not a very new problem. In the 1930s most of the states in this country, and all but one province in Canada, gave up their county institutions. Iowa and Kansas sent large numbers of their people out of institutions and into nursing homes and community centers. We did not hear too much about it at the time, but I recall that it was rather a serendipitous thing that two states—perhaps I should include Wisconsin also—held on to their county institutions and later on had fairly decent places for these people to go.

The other comment I want to add is that the situation varies from place to place. We hear a great deal of discussion about the terrible situation that arises from sending patients out into the community. In Philadelphia we ran into an extremely interesting phenomenon. Before the patients arrived in the community we had been warned that they were not wanted, and evidence to prove that it is a serious matter to send patients away from the hospital had been offered. Philadelphia happens to have extraordinarily ample psychiatric resources because of its long history as a psychiatric center, and its fine medical schools and all the other institutions like Pennsylvania Hospital in the relatively small city of only 2 million people. Thus we were able, as the statistics of various community research projects are now showing, to send large numbers of patients out into the community; but we did not do so until the system of follow-up was very carefully worked out and the operation had been really very well planned. It has been a significantly successful large-scale movement, but I suggest that the maneuver of sending patients out is not so much one of releasing them as it is one of finding them an improved place in which to live. It is so easy to forget how we cursed the back wards of the state hospitals; as soon as the patients left everyone said how wonderful the back wards of the state hospital were, and called for the patients to be sent back to them.

One other comment—I spent 15 years as a child in China. I grew up looking around the communities inside of a relatively small city where there was a fair amount of growth, although the trees gave it a country air. It was very common to see obviously psychotic people wandering around, picking up sticks and making little bundles and doing this and that. The extraordinary quality of feeling Chinese people have for the mentally ill is, I think, something that we should accept. I do not know its history but I strongly suspect that the traditions of Confucianism and the re-spect for the elderly, no matter what shape they are in, are largely responsible for the tolerance of older people, many of whom are obviously neurotic because of the old age they achieve there.

DR. KETY: What I am going to say changes the subject some-what. The question is asked whether I have an opinion on the lactate-pyruvate ratios in aerobic and anaerobic types of glucose metabolism in schizophrenic patients as suggested by Dr. Gott-lieb's research. Froman and Gottlieb have been studying this for 10 or 15 years. Although a number of people have tried, I am not aware that anyone has succeeded in confirming independently that the serum of schizophrenics has a special capacity of altering the lactate-pyruvate ratios of chicken red cells incubated with non-schizophrenic plasma. Nevertheless, Dr. Froman has continued to carry on this work and has reported increasingly purer and in-creasingly well defined characteristics of whatever it is that he finds in the plasma of the schizophrenics. Now the best studies I know that attempted to replicate this were studies done by Ryan and Durell. They were able after a while to replicate one part of

Froman's finding that the plasma of some people did in fact alter the lactate-pyruvate ratio of red cells, and they found out that this was associated with a certain amount of hemolysis of the red cells. They pursued this and found that there was a hemolytic antibody in these plasmas that was perhaps related to heterophile antibodies and/or to one of the antibodies generated by hepatitis in the past. But although they found that some people had this and some did not, and that those who did continued to have it over time, they were unable to associate this especially with schizophrenia. In a large scale study at Rockland State Hospital they found this in some of the patients, but just as frequently in nonschizophrenic as in schizophrenic patients, so until there is further evidence to support the notion that this has something to do with schizophrenia I would think that it is a nonspecific factor, related perhaps to chronic hospitalization, infectious mononucleosis, or hepatitis in the individual's past.

DR. ROMANO: I should like to ask the members of the panel and also Dr. Kramer what their predictions would be concerning the possible genetic pool of schizophrenia in the future in view of the increasing extramural presence of schizophrenic men and women, increasing fertility, and the fact that the birthrate of the psychotic population is approaching that of the nonpsychotic. We must keep in mind that according to current data, the risk—that is, the 8 per 8,000 of normal population—is increased by 10 for the child of a schizophrenic parent and multiplied 40 times with dual mating. What, then, are their predictions concerning possible changes of general psychopathology in the genetic pool, particularly in respect to schizophrenia (and perhaps creativity) with this changing demography?

DR. KETY: That's an interesting question, one which many people have thought about for some time. In fact, people have argued that, if schizophrenia exists to such a high proportion in the population that nearly 1 percent of the population is affected some time in their lives, how has it persisted to that extent over all these years unless along with the mental disorder there were some other characteristics that tended to preserve it and continue it in the genetic pool?

I think the crux of the question—and this will also help to answer Dr. Romano's question—is that this applies only when there is a very strong correlation between the genotype and the phenotype. That is, were every person who has the genetic tendency to do so to become schizophrenic, this would be a problem; but our studies seem to suggest that what is genetically transmitted is not schizophrenia itself but a predisposition to schizophrenia, and that few of those with the genetic predisposition actually become schizophrenic because of the requirement not only of the genetic predisposition but of some special constellation of environmental factors also. If that is the case, then increasing the fertility of the phenotypes will not increase the pool as markedly—although it will increase it somewhat—as if all the gene types were phenotypes. There are already enough genotypes in the population. Among us here are many who are genotypic schizophrenics but who have not become schizophrenic. And we are transmitting the genes all the time anyway. Therefore, what happens to the relatively small number of persons who are called schizophrenic, or hospitalized as such, will not affect the pool size as much. Furthermore, I imagine that better education and eugenic thinking may tend to cause people who know they are schizophrenics to reduce the number of their children voluntarily. So I think the equilibrium will probably be maintained without any very great increase taking place.

DR. SABSHIN: Dr. Kety made a point that I would have made— the assumption that a genotype leads to a phenotype. This, I think, is still incorrect; at least I hope it is, since this conclusion leaves room for a good deal of pluralism in the concept of schizophrenia. The best evidence certainly does seem to indicate a constellation of causes that includes social and psychological factors. Perhaps we could ask the question, "What happens if those social and psychological factors that are still unknown, really, interact in higher numbers? Will there be a greater shift of genotype to phenotype?" I was not altogether sure what you meant by referring to "creativity" in the last part of your question, but I assume that adding the Langian theory to other theories might establish some connection with schizophrenia. Did you mean that?

DR. ROMANO: No. Both the Iceland study and Heston's work show an increased incidence of creativity among the progeny of schizophrenics.

DR. SABSHIN: The Iceland study and another study indicate that there has been an increase in incidence of creativity in schizophrenia?

DR. ROMANO: In the children of schizophrenics.

DR. SABSHIN: I won't field that one!

DR. KETY: I think that's quite so. I know the Heston study indicated not only that the children of schizophrenics who were reared in other environments had a higher tendency to schizophrenia, but that some evidence of greater creativity among them seemed apparent. We have been attempting to evaluate that in the population we have been studying in Denmark. We have no data on it yet and so I cannot comment, but the observation has certainly been made in the literature.

DR. ROSENBERG: I should like to make two observations as a guest historian. First, the conclusion and consensus that have just been described for us in terms of the relationships between hereditary predisposition and the kinds of environmental stress that result in mental illness are precisely what most psychiatrists believed in—and expressed in almost the same words—from about 1810 to 1900. Second, of course schizophrenic individuals would be more likely to have children who showed creativity—what might have been called genius in the 19th century. This is hardly a novel observation; indeed, it is the subject of several books now receded into the distant past, or at any rate it figures only in the intellectual history of the 19th century, although it seems to have been confirmed by recent studies.

An additional kind of observation I'd like to make is a question, if you like. Dr. Sabshin pointed out in the statistics what seemed to be a surprising lack of interest in the relationship between social research and the discussion of the social factors in the etiology of mental illness. What was very striking to me in this same 10-year period that he studied was the discontinuity between the concerns of the profession and the concerns of the community with which the profession must, if possible, peacefully coexist, as evidenced not in the professional literature but in what was read by the educated and enlightened layman—the common reader, as Virginia Woolf called him. (Let's call him the *New York Review of Books* reader and make it more operational.) The most striking thing about psychiatry has been the discussion—we won't call it analysis—of the relationship between social factors and mental illness. Now I am not saying that psychiatrists are right or wrong, and, as I have said, whether this is a question is up to you, but the discrepancy certainly struck me very forcefully when I heard the statistics Dr. Sabshin gave us.

DR. SABSHIN: To respond to the two points Dr. Rosenberg has made—first, I do agree that those who forget the past really relive it; and yet I would draw a distinction between the concepts of 1810–1900 and present views inasmuch as the concept of dementia praecox belongs in that earlier period. It implied a rather gloomy prognosis. I would not underestimate the difference between that particular concept (along with the amalgam you described) and the notions of today. I think there is significance in that change. The articles in the literature of the last ten years have largely, in my judgment, emphasized psychological reality. I would make the distinction between psychological and social reality, even though we tried to indicate that there are gray areas between the two. The territories between the two have not been very clear, as, I submit, papers in the journals demonstrate. I should also try to point out that the distinction between opinion and data objectively demonstrated in research is extraordinarily slight in this area. To some extent those papers that you described would still be social. Often our reflection of aspects of feeling are less than firm in terms of hard data but are more nearly the reflections of opinion. I want to make that distinction.

Second, I think there is an artifact in the kind of studies I reported; I am sure you understand that the use of publications as criteria for evaluation of certain trends needs to take into account the time lag between the accomplishment of work and its being reported in print. Being mindful of all that, I do think, however, that you make a very nice point of discrepancies between actual high-level research and reports that appear in the public press.

DR. KRAMER: Again this may refer to some numbers that I have been able to put together from some published studies; whether or not the gene pool will reflect certain things may be looked at also in these kinds of computations. From studies we now have one can expect that about 4 to 5 percent of every cohort of 100,000 births occurring in the United States today will at some point in the lifetime develop schizophrenia, if we accept current diagnostic criteria. This would suggest that a cohort of, say, 4 million births per year could yield quite a large number of schizophrenics and have some implication for the need to plan various services.

Now also, if you will look at the number of births in the United States per year, which is in the order of 4 million, and if you assume, for example, that some unknown proportion of mothers, perhaps 10 to 20 percent, may be seriously disturbed—whether by schizophrenia or some other kind of disorder—you can predict that a large number of children will be born into families in which there is a serious problem of social disturbance of one kind or another. Such problems can have impact on the psychosocial development of the child, his health status, and a variety of other things.

This situation will require some interrelationship of the psychiatric profession with the child health profession, obstetrics and gynecology, well-baby clinics, etc., whereby there should be a greater emphasis on ways in which one might indeed foresee and forestall some problems that will threaten the children. One of the tables I gave you—I think the one that gives the age distribution of the number of people under care in at least the facilities that report to us (table 3, p. 101) —shows something in the order of 900,000 to 1 million females in the reproductive ages of life, say 18 to 44, under care in at least one of these kinds of services. With the increasing use of psychotropic drugs for depression you might have antidepressant lithium carbonate, for example. There is need for considerable interaction, it seems to me, with the obstetrics-gynecologists and pediatricians, etc., to see what can be done to get a closer liaison in the way in which available knowledge concerning the care and treatment of psychiatric disorders is being applied to this particular population. This is especially true on the basis of knowledge being accumulated that suggests that the marital patterns and reproductive rates of the mentally ill are approaching those of the general population. This situation indicates other problems that should, I think, be looked at in connection with psychiatry's relationship to the greater realm of medicine, social services, etc. I would hope that steps might be taken to optimize the application of available knowledge in order to prevent whatever problems we can prevent.

DR. MATHIS: One question from the floor to the panel in general is, How do we evaluate the approaches we talked about today?

DR. KOLB: It seems to me that if we look at the efforts of evaluation over the last 25, 35, or 45 years, there has been a progressive development due to the new designs that are being applied. I feel greatly encouraged by the materials that are coming out of our social-psychiatric groups, and also by the recognition that a number of psychiatric teams are willing to expose themselves to evaluative teams not involved in providing the treatment. In other words, in a sense we are going to get two objective evaluations of the psychotherapeutic process. Most of the evaluative instruments do not include any notice whatsoever of the subjective state of man, but most of us who are treating patients certainly listen to what the patient says to indicate his internal state, and we also recognize sometimes that the establishment of a person in a position others see as socially conforming or adaptive is not necessarily helpful to him. The real crux of the change is the internal subjective change that indicates to the individual that he is well.

DR. MATHIS: With all due regard to our good pharmaceutical men, who always support this sort of program, I once noticed in southern New Jersey that the drug most commonly prescribed on the charts was the one touted by the detail man who appeared last. I wonder, Dr. Kety, is there a better way of evaluating the biological approaches?

DR. KETY: Well, of course in the case of schizophrenia and affective disorders the pharmacological agents have been better evaluated than any of the other therapies that have been tried, in terms of research design, placebo control, double-blind, Latin square design, etc. That is a good thing, but it isn't necessarily because the pharmacologists or the psychopharmacologists are smarter than any of the others; it is just that it is easier to do a controlled study in which the therapy is a nice, encapsulated thing as opposed to social or psychoanalytic therapy, which one cannot easily encapsulate and standardize. But there really is not much of a problem in terms of evaluating the pharmacologic agents, and I think the reason that they have become so commonly prescribed and so readily recognized as valuable has simply been that these controlled trials have been confirmed by the clinical observations of the physicians who have used these agents.

DR. KOLB: They have become so commonly accepted also because some of the people who do not really feel better after taking them tell other people they do, in response to their apparent expectation.

DR. SABSHIN: I think there has been progressive development.

First, the importance of getting evaluative studies needs to be acknowledged. That still remains to be accomplished in some quarters. I think we agree well in circumstances involving gross pathology and its alteration, whether this means the patient's being able to leave the hospital or not. Hospitalization rates, for all their weaknesses, are, I think, still good criteria. I agree with Dr. Kety that in respect to psychopharmacology evaluative efforts have been better organized and more coherent, but they still have some of the limitations Dr. Kolb mentions. It appears to me that in some areas, most notably in psychoanalytic treatment and psychodynamic therapy, there may be a need to objectify the subjective nature of the response. In the area of psychopharmacology the reverse appears to be true.

It is also relevant, I think, to at least some of the comments I want to make that one of the major conceptual problems of evaluation is the issue of epidemiological studies of the healthy population as compared with the sick. It is difficult to evaluate outcome studies in the absence of the undergirding data. It will provide us with half the control populations to compare with those we treat. So one of the important developments in the future, in my judgment, would be to move toward those different kinds of approaches to make such control data more available. This does not deny the need for subjective data. I think at the beginning we start with some things that might be more than justifiable, and hope that we can find a balance in between.

The Role of Psychiatry in Society

Introduction

David R. Hawkins, M.D.

IT is with a mixture of pleasure and sadness that I chair this session of our conference—pleasure in the rich intellectual feast we have already had, pleasure in the good colleagueship of the participants in this event, and anticipatory pleasure in looking forward to today's papers and discussions; sadness in knowing that we are coming to the end of this exciting and productive exchange.

Having learned about the past, we have the task today of looking at psychiatry's role in the present and the future. Heretofore we have heard from our own colleagues in psychiatry, with the exception of Professor Dain. This morning we are asking observers of the human scene who see it from several different perspectives to tell us how we look from without. As I look at the titles of the papers I am struck with the emphasis on problems. We will hear about the crisis in psychiatric legitimacy; we will hear about some of the difficulties in our relationship with the law; and the panel discussion will raise questions about the future role of psychiatry, and its viability in the days ahead.

One of the questions that will certainly be faced by the panel today—and one that our profession certainly faces at the present moment—is the question, What is psychiatry? It was not much of a specialty at the time Eastern State Hospital opened in 1773, but I suspect that the keepers and all those people who looked after the mentally ill had little doubt about what their role in society was. Today, how do we know what we should do? In spite of the fact, as John Romano has pointed out, that psychotherapy has been a function of society for all of recorded history, and presumably for some time before that, and that Imhotep and Aesculapius and others were aware of much that goes into comprehensive psychological care, I think we might say that in many ways psychiatry is a very new discipline. In terms of its present dimensions, the roles of the people involved, and its accumulation of research of its own, psychiatry must be thought of as the newest of medical disciplines. We have heard about the phenomenal growth of our field over the last few years, and, of course, this brings problems. We have grown so fast and in so many ways we do not know where we are or where we are going.

I believe we should ask about the influence of society on psychiatry. As we have heard already, society changes whatever profession it wants to serve it, and determines its form. I think it is quite clear that what was going on in 1773 determined the type of psychiatric care people had in those days. It also seems quite clear that we in American psychiatry now are very much a function of the society in which we live. We might, for example, suggest that the overly enthusiastic and perhaps overly credulous acceptance of psychoanalysis, "lock, stock, and barrel," reflected the American optimism and belief in environmental influence. It seems a bit sad to me to contrast our times with the 18th century, and the ground upon which the figure of psychiatry appears now with the ground of social attitudes that prevailed in 1773. That was the Age of Enlightenment: a time of great ferment about wonderful new things to do for mankind, new ideas of freedom, new notions about the way to govern ourselves politically, and an enormous concern with morality. These factors all led, at the time of the foundation of Eastern State Hospital and shortly thereafter, to the techniques of "moral suasion" that we have heard documented as having been an efficacious way of dealing with mental illness. The present hardly seems to be a time of high morality. Our leaders are attempting to do away with many human services, and psychiatry has been seen as a means to an immoral end, as in the effort to steal confidential notes from Ellsberg's psychiatrist. In 1773 people believed that science and rationality would eventually overcome all human problems, but today many people—and this includes some scientists themselves—feel that science has betrayed us.

We might ask next about the influence of psychiatry on society. This has in recent years been not inconsiderable. The development of psychoanalysis, along with other factors, has contributed to the revolution in our attitude toward sexuality and child-rearing practices. The parental role is being exercised today quite differently than in the past. Our whole view of man has been influenced by the discovery of the unconscious. Our literature can never be again what it was in the pre-Freudian era. Behavioral modification raises crucial issues of concern about the manipulation and shaping of human behavior with all the attendant ethical considerations. Research in techniques of controlling human physiology and emotions by feedback procedures has led to the common use of such devices as those that induce alpha rhythm in the electroencephalogram. Dr. Romano has referred to the do-it-yourself techniques and instant cures that have been offered to the public.

We obviously have a cart-and-horse problem. Society influences psychiatry and, in turn, psychiatry exerts a powerful influence for change in society. We must regard the whole process from a transactional point of view. We who are in the field of psychiatry share a feeling of excitement and an awareness of opportunity. New understanding of the physics of the neuronal membrane, of the chemistry and pharmacology of the central nervous system, of human development, and of communication processes—all of these advances, among many others—promise to put us in a better position to care for the mentally ill while at the same time they pose new problems. Social psychiatry holds out the promise that we will learn how to prevent mental illness, although I should point out that to date there is little that is substantive behind this promise.

However, the very breadth of our field, which now encompasses everything from the molecular point of view to the most basic social issues, makes for a certain vulnerability and confusion. I think we can appropriately ask, Where are we? Where are we going? Should we treat only organic illness? Should we deal only with problems conceptualized in the learning paradigm? Should we be a force for social change? Should we emphasize primary prevention? Or should we disappear as a profession?

A major problem is whether or not we should try to speak *as a profession*. If we should, how does a profession such as ours go about the job of speaking with a clear and single voice? We have talked to one another about crucial problems at this meeting, but we are frustrated by the notion that perhaps we can do little without the backing of society at large. If we are to continue to advance we will need funds for facilities, for training, for research, for new manpower. How do we engage society as a whole in this effort? Is the education and influencing of the public an appropriate professional task?

I hope that our speakers today will have some words of wisdom about some of these issues. I am sure that in any case they will sharpen our thinking about them.

10. The Crisis in Psychiatric Legitimacy Reflections on Psychiatry, Medicine, and Public Policy

Charles E. Rosenberg, PH.D.

A TTEMPTING to define the term *psychiatry* is as difficult as it is enlightening. Psychiatry can be defined simply as a medical specialty with attendant forms of certification and accepted practice. But this is a minimal conception; in its most comprehensive meaning psychiatry is a social function, not a specialized group of physicians and their practice. The broader definition implies the response of society and its institutions to the needs of those who either see themselves as "mentally ill" or are so regarded by others, and involves all would-be healers of the mind and emotions —psychiatrists, clinical psychologists, psychiatric social workers, pediatricians and gynecologists, as well as practitioners of the most ephemeral and opportunistic psychotherapies. The gap between the limited and the comprehensive definitions of psychiatric responsibility begins itself to suggest the dimensions of the problems faced by contemporary psychiatry—problems so grave that our very public awareness of them implies a crisis in psychiatry's social legitimacy.

While American psychiatry shares all the dilemmas faced by medicine in general it must also confront a number of difficulties peculiar to itself. First, psychiatry has been—and is being—shaped by social values and needs and consequent decisions of social policy to a far greater degree than most other specialties in medicine. A second area of stress concerns the relationship between psychiatry and medicine in general. Discontinuities within the internal structure of the psychiatric community itself contribute to a third kind of problem. All three relationships—to society and its needs, to medicine, and among the several groups that make up psychiatry—are ambiguous and labile, yet they are rooted in history and tenaciously articulated in present attitudes and institutional arrangements. They will not easily be altered.

From its 19th-century beginnings as a distinct specialty, psychiatry has been shaped by decisions made outside the medical profession. The creation of asylums, for example, can hardly be interpreted as a medical decision based on a new consensus of professional opinion. Yet the establishment of such institutions created a group of physicians whose concerns centered more and more exclusively on asylum administration, and on problems of human behavior. The first title of the American Psychiatric Association was the Association of Superintendents of American Institutions for the Insane. Psychiatry was very much a specialty organized in response to a specific social need rather than the logical institutional expression of an expanding body of knowledge or the crystallization of particular techniques. Within the past generation we have seen the internal institutional structure of psychiatry, and even its intellectual framework, repeatedly affected by government policy decisions. Pressing needs after the Second World War, for example, led to the use of Veterans Administration hospitals and federal funds for psychiatric training. More recently, federal commitment to something called the community mental health center has had broad implications for the internal organization and personnel of psychiatry. Similarly, recent trends toward deinstitutionalization reflect, among other things, shifts in economic and social priorities and perceptions side by side with advances in pharmacology, and a changing intellectual consensus within psychiatry.

The term *social policy* implies conscious decisions—more and more in the 20th century those made at the level of state and federal government. But, as we are well aware, such decisions are a consequence of more general social phenomena, as, for example, attitudes toward aging, deviance, and ethnicity—as well as more fundamental structural changes like those involved in urbanization, industrialization, and consequent shifts in social values and ideology. I enumerate such factors not to shroud the discussion in a haze of diffuse and plausibly profound words, but because psychiatry relates to such structural factors somewhat differently than does medicine generally. For with the growth of technology and science a good many areas in clinical medicine have been provided with some understanding of pathological mechanisms and therapeutic resources which define at least some aspects of the clinical interaction between the physician and particular patients.

The discovery of insulin and its subsequent synthesis, for example, provides a relatively well defined therapeutic framework within which emergent cases of diabetes are managed. Yet social and economic factors play a role even in this relatively distinct and treatable condition; a particular patient may be poor and isolated or perhaps a Christian Scientist, or his physician may fail to make the proper diagnosis. Each clinical entity—and medicine's technical means for dealing with it—creates a somewhat different configuration of necessity and available therapeutic options. Thus quite a different assortment of social and economic variables structures the treatment of a particular case in which renal dialysis might be needed. In this instance, of course, such factors play a greater role than they normally would in cases of diabetes, but in both these examples the technical means at hand and insight into pathology and physiology define the parameters within which clinical decisions are made.

Psychiatry can only rarely stand on such firm ground. We still debate the fundamental basis of the most common psychiatric diagnoses and their relationship to belief systems and the realities of social structure. The contrast with most somatic ills is clear enough; if there are indeed biological mechanisms underlying even the most marked psychiatric syndromes we cannot as yet define them; if there are not, we are equally unable to demonstrate their absence; if their etiology should depend on some particular interaction of constitutional endowment and environmental stress we cannot define that relationship in more than the vaguest of terms. Every aspect of psychiatry, from its most general social conditions to the level of individual interaction between physician and patient, is inevitably shaped by extramedical factors —with comparatively few defining technological boundaries.

Of course, every area within medicine is to some extent shaped by such considerations; who is to pay for medical care, for example, and who is to regulate and certify hospitals and how they are to do it. Almost every visible 20th-century social trend relates in some way to clinical medicine. We have seen, for example, how the management of sickle-cell anemia has begun to reflect a growing black activism; we have seen the women's movement add a novel element to debate over the surgical treatment of breast cancer. But differences over mastectomy or screening for sickle-cell anemia do not alter our views of cell physiology; these debates seem merely tactical when compared to the way in which contemporary criticisms of psychiatric theory and practice have decried its most fundamental assumptions. Methodologically oriented critics have dismissed that diffuse yet generally cumulative consensus which constitutes dynamic psychiatry as being arbitrary, insusceptible of proof, and wilfully quasi-theological; social activists have attacked it as the ideology of an antihuman status quo. In the past 15 years we have seen the concept of mental illness itself assailed as an ideological construct more useful in enforcing the values of society and expressing its inability to tolerate deviance than in expressing the data of empirical observation.

As a result of such repeated criticism we have become increasingly conscious of the possible social content of psychiatric diagnoses—of the necessary tentativeness of even the most widely used diagnostic categories. We have at the same time become more conscious of the ways in which social values and structure and consequent ideological needs affect individual behavior through their shaping of role options, including those of the patient and the psychotherapist. We have become conscious, too, of the problematical quality of most cognitive therapies—not to speak of the more theoretical formulations drawn from such clinical interactions. Not surprisingly, contemporary psychiatric theory has become increasingly eclectic and hesitant. And, as we have tried to suggest, these shifts reflect not only changes in the medical and behavioral sciences, but—equally important—a changed temper in our intellectual life generally. Psychiatry could not well escape that critical mood which has questioned—among other concerns—the nature of traditional sex roles, our courts and prisons, and denounced three-centuries-old attitudes about the relationship between man and nature.

Yet despite such repeated criticisms, despite the fact that much of its theoretical foundations are still based on the exegesis of clinical intuitions, despite the fact its therapeutic means are problematic and ill defined, psychiatry must still deal with the clinical burdens of a society which "produces" vast number of individuals whose behavior is stigmatized by that society as mental illness. It must deal as well with even greater numbers suffering emotional pain and varying degrees of incapacity—behavior and emotions which many of us have come to interpret in terms of disease process.* We are no more willing, many of us, to suffer the pain of depression or anxiety than that of some more readily localized and meliorable physical ailment; in our society neither stoicism nor traditional religious viewpoints seem ordinarily to provide a context of meaningfulness for such ills of the soul. Health has come to imply the absence of emotional as well as physical pain and disability, and the physician has been defined—not entirely without his participation—as the individual best suited to deal with it. Society has, in other words, shaped over the past century and a half a special role for the psychiatrist, has provided him with a limitless abundance of clinical material—without at the same time providing him with a generally agreed-upon body of etiological and therapeutic knowledge.

Because the specialty of psychiatry has so diffuse a responsibility and possesses so little limit-defining knowledge, it is prone to border disputes; its status is critically dependent on its medical identity. Even if the formal logic and institutional appropriateness of this relationship remain problematical, its social necessity is unquestionable. Psychiatrists benefit from the status and autonomy society grants physicians—a status which may indeed serve a therapeutic role in particular doctor-patient relationships.

Yet the relationships between contemporary medicine and contemporary psychiatry are ambiguous throughout. The problem begins with medical education itself. Few will deny that the standard medical education which, despite a generation of reform, has been stubbornly resilient, is not ideally suited to the needs of those aspiring to become psychiatrists. Of course, there are the familiar justifications: the ability to differentiate genuinely functional ills from possible somatic alternatives, the assimilation of a

* We have no way of knowing or understanding the possible relationship between the reality of society's structure, values, and emotional demands, and the production of such symptoms. Thus the continuing historical and social debate as to the changing incidence and pattern of mental illness; we have, for example, no firm evidence that the incidence of felt mental illness and emotional pain is necessarily greater now than it was in the 18th or 12th or 5th centuries. We have similarly no evidence to indicate that the gravely ill were treated somehow more humanely, their experience seen as simply another dimension of the human condition. Our ignorance, of course, has implied no slackening in the vigor of the debate surrounding such problems; the relationship to a growing criticism of psychiatry, to a fashionable antirationalism, illustrates with clarity the ongoing relationship between psychiatric thought and the shifting intellectual winds of the society in which the discipline of psychiatry exists.

certain detached concern. (And the expansion of drug therapy has somewhat revitalized the argument for a conventional medical education.) But these contentions have come to seem a bit shop-worn. A justification heard with increasing frequency in recent years contends that traditional clinical training is an appropriate prerequisite for psychiatric practice in its inculcation of the responsibility implicit in the physician's control over life and death.* This claim, even if valid, is surely a marginal justification for a five-year commitment.

Another ambiguity relating to the identification of psychiatry with medicine centers on the claim of medicine to exclusive control of therapeutics. Insofar as psychiatry has voiced a similar claim, it has had a rather hollow ring; for neither available manpower nor therapeutic resources enable psychiatry to undertake realistically the exclusive care—and control—of all those defined as mentally ill. The state hospital, for example, with its formal legitimacy resting ultimately on its status as a medical institution and thus on the status and autonomy of the medical profession, illustrates dramatically the problematical nature of such identifications. It is not simply as a result of contemporary social and intellectual ferment that we entertain a crisis of what might well be called psychiatric legitimacy. The crisis also reflects the gap between the demands of medical exclusivity and the inability of psychiatry to provide either understanding or relief consistent with the pretentiousness of such demands.

And, as a matter of fact, society recognizes these realities in its unwillingness to grant holders of the medical degree exclusive control over the treatment of those who suffer emotional pain and disability. Organized psychiatry, on its part, fails to regulate effectively either its own members or other holders of medical certification who may choose to practice some form of psychotherapy.** Thus the unending production of would-be psycho-

---

* Even if contemporary biochemical insights prove fruitful in bringing understanding of schizophrenia, let us say, it is not at all clear that the physician's clinical preparation constitutes an appropriate training for such new orientation.

** Of course, general medicine has similarly failed to regulate the ethics and standards of practice of physicians, and this in many cases in which definitions of acceptable practice are more easily agreed upon. The profession has been more successful, however, in curtailing the activities of individuals who do not hold the medical degree.

therapies—under both lay and medical auspices—unregulated by either the profession or the state.

Most professions are marked by sharp distinctions between the elite and average practitioner. In the sciences and in medicine, the growing specialization and autonomy of careers oriented to basic science have only sharpened such distinctions. In psychiatry, however, the distance between elite and other practitioners is structured rather differently than in most other fields of applied science.

Historically speaking, there have been two principal styles and loci—and thus, origins—of psychiatry in the United States. One was developed out of a growing medical response to patients sufficiently ill or aged or "difficult" to require hospitalization; the other grew out of the work of physicians who treated the still-functioning though symptom-bearing patient outside of institutional settings. This distinction has existed for a century. The late-19th-century neurologist, with his prestigious private practice and earnest worship of European authority, practiced quite a different brand of psychiatry from that of the hospital-oriented curator of severely ill and often economically deprived hospital patients. Though it would be naive to contend that these categories have remained absolute and unchanged since the late 19th century, they still reflect a persistent dichotomy in psychiatric practice.

In some way, indeed, the differences are greater now than at the beginning of the century. Not only is the state hospital a locale of low status in which to practice psychiatry; it is, in general, a place where a different kind of psychiatry is practiced. In the years before World War I, ambitious young psychiatrists still frequently served in hospital positions, partly because of a lack of other available institutional niches, partly because of the intellectual concern about the psychoses and their then-still-hoped-for elucidation through pathological and biochemical approaches. (And the state and municipal hospitals were, of course, also populated by victims of organic syndromes.) With the increasing numbers of teaching and clinical positions becoming available in university medical centers, and the parallel growth in the intellectual relevance of dynamic views, the state hospitals grew progressively less attractive to many able and well-educated young psychiatrists. In the years before the First World War, moreover, it was the spiritual—and in some cases institutional—descendants of the late-19th-century neurologists who provided leadership in the adoption of dynamic psychiatry and its therapeutic implications. Advocates of this orientation and their institutional successors have since World War II consistently achieved the highest status in the profession, written most influentially, and occupied leading positions in our most prominent medical schools.

As one consequence among many others, many of the major figures in 20th-century American psychiatry have been students of the neuroses and personality disorders, not of the most severe and incapacitating conditions. (This is a pattern of interest which reflects the continuity between the neurologist's office and sanitarium practice of the late 19th century and that of the dynamically oriented psychiatrist of the mid-20th.) Not surprisingly then, much of our century's most influential psychiatric writing has consisted of general statements about the human condition, in the form of hypothetical etiologies of particular personality types and related modes of behavior. Such works have been as relevant to the educated community generally as to the narrower constituency of medical men and psychiatrists. Rather less attention has been paid to the great and dismayingly intractable clinical burdens of age, grave illness, and deviance which have traditionally filled our state hospitals. Such tendencies toward differentiation in practice and the preoccupations of research have only exacerbated distinctions within that group of physicians who term themselves psychiatrists; the channels of communication have functioned fitfully at best.*

If we see psychiatry as a function rather than as a group of appropriately certified practitioners, a number of other structural problems become apparent. One lies in the fact that physicians without formal psychiatric training habitually practice ad hoc "psychiatry." We all know pediatricians and gynecologists, for

---

* And there is a further irony. Almost all 20th-century psychiatrists have been clinicians (at least until they became administrators). Yet this identity as clinicians has not helped create a community of interest. In addition to the fact that the clinical concerns of both groups have differed, the concern with clinical situations and the elaboration of clinical intuitions created (or, perhaps more accurately, preserved) an ethos inhospitable to more positivistic standards of scientific proof— an ethos grounded in a need to find and accept explanatory formulae, almost a necessity for physicians who must actually deal with patients.

example, who casually dispense psychiatric dicta with their infant formulae or birth-control pills. This segment of what might be called psychiatric practice is little amenable to control and far removed from the work and attitudes of the elite within psychiatry.

The intellectual relationship between the several levels of practice and investigation is even more tenuous in psychiatry than in most other areas of medicine, although it is, of course, problematical to an extent in every area of applied science. The most isolated or provincial internist or general practitioner routinely employs drugs the physiological activity and chemical structure of which he understands little. But the laboratory man who ascertained the activity of a particular substance, the technicians who developed and tested it, have communicated with the practitioner through a cultural artifact. This species of communication has—with the comparatively recent exception of the psychoactive drugs—hardly existed in psychiatry. The psychiatric elite has in general given the state hospital physician, the pediatrician or urologist, or the general practitioner little in the way of discrete and portable artifacts. Even if one assumes a certain validity for the insights of the dynamic tradition, they are neither easily communicated nor easily utilized, though they are easily vulgarized.

The last half-century, with its generally increasing public acceptance of psychiatry, has only intensified the profession's dependence on lay values and policy decisions. In no area has this been more clearly demonstrated than that of society's search for the means of dealing with deviance. Psychiatry cannot win for winning; the more confidence laymen have placed in psychiatry and psychiatric procedures, the more importunate are the demands made upon it, and inevitably the greater the gap between expectation and performance. American psychiatry, not without the participation of certain of its own spokesmen, has become to an extent committed to finding solutions for such perceived problems as juvenile delinquency, drug addiction, criminality, and variant sexual behavior. Psychiatry has in this sense become a kind of residual legatee for the attempt to solve some of society's most intractable problems—and not without a certain logic and even idealism informing the series of attitudes and decisions which brought about this involvement.

The situation is again ambiguous. Many individuals who behave in ways perceived as antisocial do exhibit symptoms of personality disorder. It is abundantly clear as well that society's other institutions—preventive and remedial—have shown themselves consistently incapable of dealing with such individuals. Thus a measure of social commitment as well as a necessary faith in the efficacy and meaningfulness of their own clinical orientation has, in the past half-century, convinced many psychiatrists that they should play some role in society's attempts to deal with such problems. (A normal component of personal ambition and pride of profession has presumably played a role as well.)

Thus the often vigorous demands for a greater role in the adjudication and treatment of the criminal offender were made by certain forensic psychiatrists in the first half of this century. It was natural for such psychiatrists to endorse or articulate rhetorical onslaughts against the "obscurantism" of the law and lawyers—and the harsh and seemingly dysfunctional punishments meted out to criminal offenders who might be mentally irresponsible; legal ideas and institutions seemed to reflect the nature of human motivation inadequately. But a half-century of such debate and a few hesitant experiments have brought few results. State and federal legislators and administrators have been unwilling generally to underwrite even the widespread experimental application of individual psychotherapeutic techniques—and it has become increasingly clear that even if they had, beneficial results could not well have been guaranteed. The demands of the psychiatric establishment that it participate in judging and treating the criminal offender seem more and more remote in intellectual history as would-be reformers increasingly concern themselves with the nature of penal institutions and the structural realities and values of the society that produces the individuals incarcerated in them. The gift of social responsibility is always dubious insofar as it implies an embittering gap between expectations and performance.

Nevertheless, some of my best friends are psychiatrists. I have several explanations for this, some more complimentary than others, but I have decided that it is principally because of our parallel marginality to the world of medicine. Psychiatrists are more likely than other medical specialists to take an interest in the history of their subdiscipline; there may even be a kind of truth in the hostile whimsy that such historical interest reflects the fact that psychiatrists practice medicine as it was practiced a century or more ago.

But insofar as this is true it should evoke sympathy rather than condemnation. All societies need physicians to deal with those conditions that cause pain and disability and are defined as illness. The mid-19th-century physician could neither cure nor explain tuberculosis or typhoid, but he had to treat them nevertheless. They would not go away, nor will those grave forms of disability our society calls psychoses, or those less disabling ones that cause "only" depression and anxiety.

Indeed, the contemporary psychiatrist is in some ways in a position even more difficult than that of his mid-19th-century predecessor. There are two reasons for this. One is the way in which psychiatry has, as we have argued, inherited a bewildering variety of social problems. The psychiatric profession obviously cannot make—or plausibly even formulate—policy in regard to racial discord, crime, or optimum modes of schooling, yet it bears in the minds of at least some Americans a certain burden of responsibility (in some minds, ironically, a responsibility for curing, in others for somehow causing such problems). There is a second and far more fundamental difficulty. Even if developing scientific knowledge should restructure the doctor-patient relationship in severe conditions of mental disability as insulin has done in the treatment of diabetes and antibiotics in the treatment of pneumonia, it seems most unlikely that we will find analogous understanding for all those conditions we call neurotic or label as personality disorders.* They are presumably modes of adjustment and thus expressions of our emotional reality; as long as our social values venerate medical and manipulative solutions and fail to provide other sources of consolation, the psychiatrist (or some other designated figure) will continue to inherit a goodly share of this burden. A major justification of medical psychiatry's legitimacy lies not in its ability to diagnose, predict and cure—nor even in its possible ethical superiority to rival schools of emotional healing—but in the very gravity and scale of the responsibility it must undertake. Psychiatry has a second claim to social legitimacy, one that upholds and justifies its continued relation-

* It should be recalled that pellagra and paresis were in this century problems for the psychiatrist.

ship with medicine: while we await the unpredictable gestation of research to tell us more of etiology and mechanisms that may underlie mania, depression, and what is called schizophrenia, psychiatry provides the principal link between laboratory and clinical research and the social reality of these ailments.* Not effectiveness, but orientation, values, and responsibility are the basis of psychiatry's legitimacy.

Criticism of the theoretical frameworks used most frequently in the past half-century to explain such conditions cannot obviate the implacable reality of the conditions themselves. And such explanatory frameworks have a certain legitimacy of their own, even if they are arbitrary and perhaps ultimately inadequate. Just as society needs someone to treat those it labels sick, such designated healers need an ideological framework with which to rationalize their ministrations. It is true that these formulations have, in the absence of limit-defining physiological and pathological data, provided an ideology that on the one hand supports the practitioner's role and status, and on the other incorporates general social norms and values.

The assumptions of certain psychiatrists may have seemed to endorse particular patterns of family, caste, and sex roles, and to be suspiciously consistent with the needs of an urban, rationalistic society unwilling to tolerate certain kinds of deviance. But it is not clear where this observation leaves us; for even if we change the assumptions of American psychiatry, we are unlikely to alter those social and individual factors that figure in the causation of mental dysfunction. A change of viewpoint may have an enlightening, but hardly a healing effect. Even if one assumes that the macrostructure of society and the not entirely unrelated microstructure of the family play some precipitating role in the

---

* This second argument can be clarified by returning to the analogy with mid-19th-century medicine. It is sometimes tempting for the historian to look with scorn upon the medical establishment of a century ago, to make its therapeutics and speculative etiologies an object of ridicule. At least the irregulars—the argument follows—the homeopaths, botanics, and eclectics who were little hindered by traditional dogma, did little to harm their patients—and they provided a cogent criticism of the contemporary medical establishment. Yet seen in perspective, the criticism of irregulars only underlines the strength of regular medicine; it was part of a world system of knowledge and accepted techniques for its acquisition and dissemination. It was this relationship to European clinical and scientific work that distinguished leaders in regular medicine, not the shortcoming of their therapeutics or their arbitrary and speculative etiologies.

etiology of mental illness, psychiatry is hardly the most important or effective institution through which society controls and defines behavior.

It may be that different arrangements within society would perhaps reduce the number of individuals who suffer emotional discomfort. *Perhaps,* indeed. But this conviction does not help the sick today, nor does it serve as an adequate rationale for the dissolution of contemporary psychiatry—or even the dissolution of the much maligned "medical model" as a framework within which to work. Individuals will continue to suffer in varying degrees from what will continue to be defined in our rationalistic society as mental illness. And most of those unable to live with their emotional selves will either turn voluntarily or be sent to psychiatrists who offer some rationalistic mode of therapy. (Behavioral and psychopharamacological techniques fit in general into this pattern.) Neither the growth of mystical and supposedly transcendent sects nor the growth of a fashionable antirationalism promises to change this view in the near future. Most Americans simply have no other emotional and cognitive frame of reference in which to place their feelings. The religious values which provided such a framework in the past seem no longer compelling to most Americans; there is no meaning, no compensation in their emotional pain. Thus the so-called medical model—for better or worse—with its implication of disease process and expectation of cure has to a certain extent replaced these older frameworks for coping with depression and anxiety.*

The opening of the 1970s finds psychiatry in a particularly eclectic and labile state. One of its strongest threads of continuity lies, ironically, in the very persistence of those structural dilemmas we have sought to describe. Unless all psychiatry should thaw, melt, and resolve itself into applied pharmacology there seems little possibility of these difficulties redefining themselves. Drug therapy itself, for example, represents a potential shift in traditional modes of psychiatric practice (and, by implication, theory as well). Yet even when it provides symptomatic relief and leads

---

* These remarks are only marginally relevant to conditions of extreme disability, some of which have known organic causes and others of which may well be found to be dependent upon some underlying physical mechanism. Even in such severe conditions, of course, social values and expectations help shape the attitudes of others toward the sufferer and, to an extent, his conception of self.

to new theoretical insights, psychopharmacology seems to support the criticism that psychiatry has failed to evaluate adequately the efficacy of its cognitive therapeutic procedures. Nor have those activist critics who see in psychiatry an agent of social control been reassured by current emphasis on drug therapy. Behavioral therapies only restate and reaffirm like ambiguities, for these newer techniques reflect not only the influence of contemporary intellectual trends but, almost simultaneously, parallel reactions to them. Drug and behavioral therapies only reformulate the persistent problems implicit in psychiatry's social location and its sensitivity to social and intellectual currents. We find ourselves in a period of unprecedented and unashamed questioning; skepticism has become our most plausible candidate for orthodoxy. And this is perhaps not too deplorable a situation.

11. A Role for Psychiatry in the Future: A Proposal

Morris S. Schwartz, PH.D.

A COMMEMORATIVE occasion has its own dynamics and its own requirements. It is a time for reflection and appraisal, for weighing the satisfactions of the past against its disappointments, for measuring the realities of the present against the ideals, for projecting optimistic hopes and thoughtful resolutions about the future, and for proffering and accepting congratulations on having survived while still performing a useful function. But, above all, for a profession these occasions afford an opportunity for provocative questioning, for uncomfortable challenges, for serious soul-searching, and for a detached look at where the profession is and where it might go. This I intend to do as a questioning outsider who has had a long association with psychiatrists. I hope that my provocations will stimulate you to engage the issues and explore solutions to the problems that seem critical to me.

Any profession must be viewed in the context of the society of which it is a part. This is especially true of psychiatry since it deals with human beings and their disturbances. For there is a dynamic reciprocal relation between the two, with the society establishing the boundaries and conditions of the kind of psychiatry that can and should be practiced, and sanctioning and legitimating that practice, and with the profession, through its practices and ideals, influencing the values and ideology of the society that supports it. Thus the relation between society and profession is an intimate one, and if we want to project a role, or change in role, for a psychiatry of the future, we must be able to identify some of the dominant themes in the society that have particular relevance for psychiatric practice. Many of these societal themes are well known to you: rapid social change, the dominant role of science and technology, value confusion, the disintegration of norms by which to judge ethical conduct, and so on.

The theme I particularly wish to address is that of *de-*

humanization—a phenomenon I see as a central destructive influence in our society, and one with which psychiatry is directly concerned. For the tendency to de-humanize the other is pervasive and deeply ingrained in our institutions. It affects the thinking, feeling, and conceptions of all of us. And it operates in subtly unconscious as well as in planned directed ways within and through these institutions. Its consequences are the erosion of our humanity, the corrosion of our emotions, and the contamination of our interpersonal relations. And the ways in which de-humanization manifests itself and the forms it takes in society are particularly relevant for psychiatry for two reasons. First, it is the antithesis of the humanitarianism that originally inspired an enlightened psychiatry and today infuses its highest achievements. And, second, it is a dominant disintegrative force of our time which influences, intertwines with, and is part of individual disturbances. Thus, I see de-humanization as a cause for, a correlate of, and a reciprocator to the individual psychological distress that is the central concern of psychiatry.

Since I shall focus on and use the concepts of de-humanization, and its opposite, humanization, as central ideas in this paper, I shall try to convey to you the way in which I define them.

I have conceptualized six forms of de-humanization. There are undoubtedly other forms and other ways of conceptualizing them. First, de-humanization can take the form of *psychosocial reduction,* in which the individual is dealt with as if he were non-existent as a psychosocial being. These are the relationships in which one's personhood or individuality is disregarded or annihilated. This form of de-humanization is characteristic of the automated workplace where the faceless worker is lost in the sea of other unrecognized entities, and of a mass society in which the anonymous consumer is seen only as a potential spending machine.

Closely related to psychosocial reduction and overlapping with it is a form of de-humanization that I call *status immersion.* Here the person is treated exclusively in terms of the function he is expected to serve or identified primarily with the status or position he occupies. It is the part one plays in the organization that is important, rather than who is playing the part. Status immersion is characteristic of bureaucracies where the expectation is that one will keep one's hierarchical place in the social order, that one will impersonally carry out orders without questioning them, that one will fulfill organizational requirements regardless of personal inclination, values, or what the situation at hand seems to call for.

Routinization is a third form of de-humanization. Where routinization prevails, the person is dealt with in stereotyped, automatic, repetitive ways, without concern for his uniqueness as a person. Routinization is common for participants in large-scale organizations in which the intention is to treat them, and they experience themselves as being responded to, in standardized, preestablished ways. The routine dominates the interaction of the participants.

A fourth mode of de-humanization I identify as *de-personing*. In this mode, persons are responded to as not quite human, as less than human, or as nonhuman. This is reflected in societal attitudes and actions toward persons who are conceived of as deviants, outsiders, or unacceptables. De-personing is embedded in the language we use about them. Homosexuals are called "perverts," mental patients are labeled "lunatics" or "maniacs," blacks are referred to as "primitives" or "niggers," and Indians are thought of as "savages."

A fifth de-humanizing form, *object-making*, is pervasive in our institutions in the business world. Here persons are used as means to profit-making ends, as tools of production, and as vehicles for material aggrandizement.

In the last form of de-humanization, which I call *reification*, persons are responded to as members of a class or as an abstract category. Thus, mental patients, the poor, the old, the worker are treated not as distinguishable individuals with a variety of idiosyncratic characteristics and attributes, but in terms of a stereotype that is attached to a single category by which they are being labeled.

By contrast, when humanization is present, one is accorded the status of fellow human being with all the entitlements pertaining thereto. The individual is recognized and respected as a unique and worthwhile person; he is accorded the right to exist as a physical and psychosocial being; he is treated as an end in himself; he is included in a common humanity; he is responded to as a totality, as a whole human being; and he is seen as one who has the potentiality for becoming other than what he is.

As I have indicated, de-humanization is a dominant disintegrative process in our time and place. It impinges upon and penetrates the lives of everyone in our society, while, by comparison, humanization takes a secondary place and plays a minor role in our institutions. The profession of psychiatry cannot isolate itself or remain aloof from this societal current, for these de-humanizing processes are a critical set of noxious conditions that contribute to, constitute, and reinforce individual disturbance and emotional distress. Thus the psychiatric profession is confronted with a choice: to continue to take existing institutions for granted and to leave attempts to change them to some other group, or to make an explicit value choice and take an active role in opposing de-humanization and in creating humane institutions.

One consequence of continuing his present stance is that the psychiatrist deceives himself into believing he is genuinely neutral with respect to societal issues. I say "deceives himself" because in the societal arena there is no value neutrality. By not taking a position and by passively accepting current institutional arrangements, the psychiatrist becomes an active contributor to, or an unconscious facilitator of, things as they are. And, as such, he perpetuates the phenomenon of de-humanization. In addition, by ignoring what contributes to and constitutes a noxious social milieu, treatment of emotional disturbance is limited, and prevention of mental distress and promotion of mental health constitute a feeble and ineffective exercise.

Thus the psychiatrist, by not confronting in his practice and theory distress-producing social and institutional phenomena and by confining his efforts to the neurophysiological, the chemical, the intrapsychic, the interpersonal, or the small-group approaches —no matter how valid they are in themselves—avoids grappling with an important contributory cause and treatment possibility. As a consequence of this restriction, the psychiatrist ordinarily treats the anxiety of the designated patient—be the patient an individual, a group, or a family—but ignores the myriad ways in which our society induces insecurity; he treats the patient's low self-esteem but ignores the recurrent social constraints and compulsions that force us into subordinate and powerless positions; he treats the person's difficulties in loving another yet ignores the social conditions that encourage him to view others as competitors or enemies; he treats the individual paranoia but ignores the institutional ways in which we are investigated to find out if we espouse dissident ideas; he treats the hostility but ignores the violence perpetrated by the society; he treats the lack of commitment but ignores the societal cynicism and the erosion of norms and values; he treats the identity crisis but ignores the societal fragmentations, discontinuities, contradictions, and lack of community that help generate them; he treats the confusion but ignores the deliberate deceptions and distortions of truth that have become customary in the political and governmental scene; finally, he treats the detachment or affectlessness, but ignores our bombardment by meaningless and inane stimuli in our mass media.

My thesis is not simply that large-scale social problems, such as war and poverty, contribute significantly to emotional distress but that these distresses are *generated every day by our institutions in the ordinary course of their normal functioning.*

We thus have a basic dilemma: by treating only the individual or the small group as if these were the exclusive source of a person's problems, the psychiatrist is ignoring a major and significant source of emotional disturbance—that is, our social system. Even if he wanted to, the psychiatrist could not be expected to grapple with *all* of these overwhelming societal dysfunctions. However, by treating only individuals, the psychiatrist does not affect the institutions of which they are a part. Yet these very institutions, if left unexamined, uncontested, and unmodified, will produce, renew, reinforce, and continue emotional distress. Still, to try to deal with these institutions all at once, and each in its totality, is an impossible task for any group. Thus we have both the apparent necessity and the apparent impossibility; how then to break out of this impasse?

I can propose some ways out of this dilemma. First, the psychiatrist needs a broader conceptual framework; the individual and his institutions must be conceptualized together and understood in their interconnectedness. Second, I propose that psychiatrists develop strategies and experiment with procedures to pursue humanization as a central value, and that this attempt to diminish de-humanization and increase humanization become his initial mode of penetrating and changing institutions that are distress-producing. I am not unmindful of the problems, difficulties, complexities, and dangers involved in this proposal, especially the problem of trying to combine analytic objectivity with an explicit value commitment. Nor am I unaware of the comfort, security, and safety that has to be relinquished to pursue both a detached interpretive mode *and* a committed action orientation. Nevertheless, I am persuaded that if psychiatrists continue to use the orientations and methods currently extant, if they avoid confronting the society, its culture, and its institutions—especially as these affect de-humanization and humanization—the basic problems of how to diminish emotional distress, prevent its occurrence, and optimize its treatment will remain unsolved. Psychiatrists will continue to pick up the wreckage and the pieces while these are being created in great profusion by institutional processes outside their control or directed effort.

It seems to me that the critical questions are: Can the psychiatrist engage in a new set of functions, combine them with old functions, and thereby create an enlarged social role for himself? Can he be both analyst of, and educator about, the psychological and social phenomena that distress him and his patients? Can he also be advocate and proponent of the ways in which he and his patients might change their social environments so as to minimize their de-humanizing qualities? Finally, can he be the activist-agent that facilitates and brings about the individual and social changes that actually foster humanization? Thus what I am proposing is to add a set of new functions to the psychiatrist's role that will focus his intellectual effort and his energy on the de-humanizing aspects of our society and their relation to, and impact upon, individuals. I am proposing that the psychiatrist make a self-conscious and deliberate choice to be an agent of humanizing social change at times and in ways that are appropriate, and in those arenas that are accessible to him. In sum, I am suggesting that the psychiatrist be a social-systems analyst and activist as well as a person or family-system analyst and activist, in order to participate in and facilitate humanizing institutional transformations in the interest of individuals.

Although the boundaries and content of this proposed role require experimentation, trial and error, groping, and caution before it "shakes down" into acceptable forms and procedures, I shall take the liberty of suggesting some possible functions in this new role. As analyst-educator, the psychiatrist might try to develop the conceptual tools, theories, and insights that would enable us to understand the relation of individual pathology to social pathology at different levels of social complexity. Here the attempt would be to identify and conceptualize the sets of intersecting and interconnecting individual, familial, institutional and societal processes that bring about emotional distress. This means that the psychiatrist would view his patients not only as distressed personalities but also as reflections of, vehicles for, transmitters of, participants in, and creators of a de-humanizing culture. In addition, he would communicate this knowledge and understanding to patients in particular and to the public in general.

I propose that he start as critic by undertaking a thoroughgoing examination of the social structures and processes in which he participates and which he supports—such as mental hospitals, prisons, courts, community health clinics, and private practice, as well as his professional organizations and practices—to identify and evaluate de-humanizing phenomena therein, and to propose and devise strategies for changing these social systems in the direction of greater humanization.

The questions the psychiatrist would confront as activist agent are: What changes might be, or must be, brought about (when, how, where, with whom, and with what means) to promote the humanizing principle? Thus, for example, he might work with patients to help them identify and understand their de-humanizing social environment, which contributes to and is part of their emotional distress. He might help them become agents of humanizing social change in their immediate social situations. In addition to maintaining an inward focus on patient dynamics, he would focus outward with the patient to help him find creative ways of changing the social conditions that occasion distress.

In addition, the psychiatrist, recognizing that emotional distress is not only an intrapsychic phenomenon but also a reflection of a socially induced collective phenomenon—and that each needs to be addressed and engaged—might work directly with and against institutions to help them re-form and restructure their organization and their functioning so that they generate more humanizing effects.

Finally, psychiatry as a profession might join with others to constitute a pressure group opposing de-humanizing societal processes and encouraging institutional humanization.

Some of these specific suggestions may sound strange and unacceptable to you; others may sound familiar and may already be part of your role. The specific suggestions are not as important as the exploration of how to expand the psychiatric role. I intend these suggestions to be beginnings for thinking about how psychiatrists might combine and integrate the functions of clinician-specialist with those of humanist-generalist and social analyst–activist–functions that are ordinarily kept separate and distinct from each other. But these are not ordinary times, nor are you grappling with an ordinary problem.

I do not underestimate the risk, the complexity, or the difficulty in transforming psychiatric work in the direction I have proposed. But it seems to me that the complexity and difficulty of understanding, dealing with, and preventing emotional distress in our society must be matched by a parallel complexity, daring, and imagination of psychiatric practice. It is this difficult task in unchartered territory that I urge on you. Already overburdened with a variety of functions, perspectives, and methods—neurochemical, psychodynamic, interpersonal, and family processual—psychiatrists might strenuously object to being saddled with an additional set of functions, asking: "Why us, and why now?" All I can answer is: "If not you, who? If not now, when?"

Bibliography

Buber, M.: *Between Man and Man.* New York: Macmillan, 1965.

———: *The Knowledge of Man.* New York: Harper Torch Books, 1965.

Gralnick, A., and D'Elia, F.: The humanizing influence of the psychiatric hospital. *Journal of the National Association of Private Psychiatric Hospitals* 2:26–29, 1970.

Ottenberg, P.: Dehumanization in social planning and community psychiatry. *American Journal of Psychotherapy* 22:585–91, 1968.

Schwartz, M.: *The Human Being as Mental Patient.* Forthcoming.

12. The Role of Psychiatry in Society
A Jurist's Viewpoint

David L. Bazelon, LL.D

YOUR conference has been devoted to an assessment of psychiatry from a number of different perspectives. My remarks this morning are simply how I see the profession of psychiatry from my window on its world — or should I say from my bench?

My message is essentially a simple one — it is that psychiatrists, especially those who work in institutions, must face the necessity for greater accountability. The future roles of psychiatry depend in large part on the public's confidence in the psychiatrist's willingness to allow scrutiny of his profession at work. In our society, part of the task of scrutinizing the expert decision-makers in a great many disciplines has fallen to the judiciary. And it is this task which the expert decision-makers in psychiatry have especially failed to appreciate or understand. I would like to share with you a very recent experience which illustrates this misapprehension of what my job as a judge is all about.

I have been inquiring into the current assessment of psychiatry through the peer review mechanism. In response, a very prominent psychiatrist (whom I shall refer to as Dr. X) accused me of, in his words, "astonishing chutzpah." Who was I to raise such questions when I lack the necessary expertise, he asked. In effect, I was told to stick to my job of being a judge. As far as he was concerned, the assessment should be left to psychiatrists who have the needed insight into the problems of the profession. No camel's nose was about to be allowed inside this sacrosanct tent. My motives were also challenged, and the final riposte was that judges could use similar assessments — in other words, we should clean out our own stables.

Dr. X seems to forget a cardinal rule of psychotherapy: be alert to patient resistance manifested on the couch by talk about others instead of about personal problems. This rule seems to apply to psychiatrists as well when the spotlight focuses on them! Dr. X is one of the leading researchers and teachers in American psychiatry, one whom I respect highly and consider a good friend. His contributions in psychiatric research and training have been enormous. It is distressing that a psychiatrist of his stature would respond in a way which is so depressingly similar to my experience with other psychiatrists in the courts. This kind of response indicates to me a serious misunderstanding of what the role of the expert is in the judicial process.

As a judge of the United States Court of Appeals in Washington, I have been exposed for the past 24 years to almost every sensitive scientific and medical question that has legal or moral implications for society. They include—to mention only a few—therapeutic abortion, the nuclear explosion at Amchitka, the safety of nuclear power plants all over the country, the pollution of air and water. I approach these issues *not* as the doctor, *not* as the physicist, *not* as the ecologist—*not* as the expert of any medical, technological, or scientific discipline. I approach these issues only as the one charged with monitoring and supervising the decisional process. This is my role in dealing with questions relevant to psychiatry, such as, for example, Who can be held morally responsible for a crime? Who can be ordered into a hospital for compulsory treatment? What kinds of treatment can be imposed involuntarily, and for how long? What is the child's right to treatment in the juvenile justice system? These questions present issues on the balance of power between the state and the individual. But the effort to strike that balance requires the knowledge and expertise of those in the behavioral sciences.

Please remember that these questions arise on petitions for a redress of grievances. This is the business—this is the stuff of the judicial enterprise. These questions may *not* properly be avoided or ignored.

It is true that many judges have more sense than to take on in depth the thornier issues of behavioral sciences posed in cases before the courts. But, maybe because I had a Jewish mother, I am more easily trapped and troubled. Perhaps I am not too *un*consciously seeking to dump my frustration onto you.

In any event, and to speak seriously, I deeply believe that over the years I have been given a unique opportunity to develop personal and, I believe, sympathetic insights into the inner workings of your profession. I have participated in countless activities in the behavioral sciences—to name only a few, membership on the

National Academy of Sciences Committee on Child Development and on the National Advisory Council of NIMH, and presidency of the American Orthopsychiatric Association. I have seen psychiatry grappling with the worst problems of our time—trying to make its expertise relevant to crime, poverty, racism, child abuse, and more. Yet my 20 years of bridge-building between the law and behavioral sciences have been stormy, at best. I have been the darling of the psychiatric establishment—receiving a Certificate of Commendation from the APA as well as being designated an honorary fellow.

More recently, as those of you who read the APA newspaper realize, I have become somewhat of a pariah and nemesis in the eyes—or should I say in the words—of its editor. No wonder then than my purported views are currently under siege in the letters to the editors published in the most recent *APA News*.

At the very beginning of my judicial career I hoped that the psychiatrists would willingly bring into the courtroom all the information available on the determinants of human behavior, and reveal what is known and (just as importantly) what is *not known* about these factors. I believed such information would not only have a significant impact on the fact-finding and value-judging tasks of the court—but would also humanize the law. Instead, psychiatrists in court quickly adopted a protective and defensive stance. They refused to submit their opinions to the scrutiny which the adversary process demands. It is remarkable how psychiatrists' current response to the public's concern about what they are doing closely parallels the defensive reaction which I observed for many years in court. The profession's refusal—or perhaps its inability—to submit its expertise to public review has generated much of the current crisis of confidence which is rapidly undermining public trust. But if strong resentment voiced by Dr. X, a distinguished leader of American psychiatry, is any indication, then surely my perspective—derived from the legal system —suggests that resistance to public scrutiny runs far deeper than I had thought possible.

What I have seen of the psychiatrist's battles with the adversary process in the courtroom is relevant for the psychiatrist's struggle in the community. Let me briefly summarize what I mean by the *adversary* process. The adversary process does not create *adversity*. (I use the term *adversity* to mean opposition and conflict.) The adversary process is merely the decisional mechanism for attempting to resolve the adversity. A court *must* make decisions, with or without sufficient knowledge. It cannot postpone decisions until the day such knowledge is available. Many might argue that, since the decision is imperfect anyway, the effort to obtain all possible information is not worth it. In the parlance of the Office of Management and Budget, the cost-benefit ratio is prohibitive. But as judges we have an awesome awareness of the great risk of rendering imperfect decisions which often entail enormous consequences for the individual and our society. Consequently I feel a tremendous responsibility to tighten rather than to relax our efforts to obtain the best information possible upon which to rest the decisions we cannot defer.

The law seeks to do this in dealing with both factual and value conflicts. In dealing with factual conflicts, we rely on an exhaustive inquiry; adversary roles are assigned to bring into the open the reality of the underlying dispute. Parties and counsel must make the best possible case for themselves, and must check and correct their adversary's material.

Specific rules have been developed to make the system both skeptical and objective. These rules presuppose that people are biased, that their testimony and opinions are inevitably shaped by their backgrounds, personalities, interests, and values. Cross-examination challenges witnesses for their veracity, accuracy, and bias. Steps are taken to select fact-finders—the jury members—who can be expected to be impartial. The legal profession is expected to be sensitive to its own conflicts of interest and to make sure that counsel does not serve more than one master .

We might be able to develop better rules to elicit facts in the courtroom and to dispel the excesses which spawn charges of hostility from those subjected to rigorous cross-examination. But although we are fully aware of its potential strengths and weaknesses, the adversary process is the mechanism we have carefully chosen and that we now rely upon to uncover as many of the relevant facts as possible.

In addition to the discovery of facts, the law also deals with competing interests and values which seem irreconcilable. In this task the common law does not seek final solutions; it recognizes the continuing nature of deep-rooted conflicts. A judge reviews and fashions criteria for resolving each case as it comes. The criteria are made known to the public in written opinions; the competing values are ventilated. Consequently, the judgments are never fixed or frozen because they can be altered in response to new information, new understanding, or new public demands. Law does not provide a wisdom unto itself. It only suggests a method for seeking wisdom. It insures that the conflicts and competing values are honestly aired rather than covered up.

The "adversary process" is thus a metaphor for what I take to be the hallmark of my world: the recognition that adversity and the conflicting values which flow from it exist, and must be treated accordingly. It seems to me this is the premise of the theory and practice of psychiatry! Conflict, whether intrapsychic or extrapsychic, exists. Psychotherapy is a process of uncovering the underlying forces that create and perpetuate these conflicts. Through such exploration the emotional discomfort and disability can begin to be resolved.

My first exposure to psychiatry inside the courtroom concerned the expert opinions which psychiatrists were asked to render in criminal trials. In the early 1950s, psychiatry and law were at a standstill on the issue of criminal responsibility—the so-called insanity defense. The traditional legal test permitted psychiatric testimony to focus on a narrow issue—whether the defendant *knew* what he was doing, and *knew* whether it was right or wrong. Strictly construed, this might mean whether he *knew* that the knife in his hand was *not* a toothbrush. The psychiatric profession was outspokenly critical of this test. The test seemed to ignore the modern dynamic theories of man as an integrated personality; it focused on one aspect of that personality—cognitive reason—as being the sole determinant of conduct. Psychiatrists publicly claimed that if the law would let them, they could give a more adequate account of psychic realities and present a vast array of scientific knowledge of human behavior.

Prominent psychiatrists also complained that the legal test compelled the doctor to decide the issue of moral responsibility, which under our legal system should be left to the jury. They insisted that psychiatrists should be allowed to address the issue of responsibility in terms relevant to their medical discipline without the distortions of the moral and legal prisms.

The law recognizes that the question of guilt or innocence is essentially a moral one. I believe—and I suspect that you would agree—that real moral judgments cannot rest on abstract philosophical principles but must derive from the facts which generate human behavior in the *real* world.

To obtain these facts in 1954 I formulated a new test of criminal responsibility in the *Durham* case. That case held that an accused is not criminally responsible if his unlawful act was the product of a mental disease or defect. *Durham* was not based on a belief that psychiatrists knew everything there was to know about behavior. Its announced purpose was to unfreeze what knowledge they did have, to irrigate a field parched by lack of information, and to restore to the jury its traditional function—to apply "our inherited ideas of moral responsibility to those accused of crime."

Psychiatric response to the new rule was enthusiastic—the profession had stated its willingness to introduce its expertise into the courtroom and here was its chance. Dr. Karl Menninger described the decision in 1954 as "more revolutionary in its total effect than the Supreme Court decision [also in 1954] regarding segregation." If the revolution which *Durham* set in motion comes with the same "deliberate speed" as the desegregation ordered by the Supreme Court, only our great-grandchildren will be able to check out Dr. Karl's appraisal.

I will not detail the laborious process which ensued in countless cases and opinions to try to fulfill the promise of *Durham*. The promise was unfulfilled. The purpose was not achieved. Yet we can learn a great deal from examining why *Durham* failed to live up to these expectations. Failure is often a more important teacher than success. We learned that despite our best efforts, psychiatrists continued to use conclusory labels without explaining the origin, development, or manifestations of a disease in terms meaningful to the jury.

Psychiatrists argued about whether a defendant had a "personality defect," a "personality disorder," a "disease," an "illness," or simply a "type of personality." How could a jury or any one else really make any sense out of this when the psychiatrists couldn't agree on the definitions? It was as if psychiatrists resorted to deliberate obscurantism to maintain an illusory elitism.

What the psychiatrist has apparently never been able to understand is that conclusory labels and opinions are no substitute for facts derived from disciplined investigation. Labeling a person "schizophrenic" does not make him so! Although the law can expect only an "educated guess," that guess is only as good as the *investigation*, the *facts*, and the *reasoning* that underlie it. It seems quite apparent to me now that the overall sterility of psychiatry's response to the *Durham* rule was due to the fact that it had made the doctor's courtroom role *much more* difficult and demanding than ever before—and therefore very much *more* threatening.

I don't believe that psychiatrists deliberately sought to sandbag the *Durham* rule, but they did find ways to sidestep its rigor by simply covering up their uncertainties, lack of investigation, and lack of knowledge. Psychiatrists refused, for example, to talk in public about the very real factors which impeded the kind of psychiatric investigation *Durham* had contemplated. After a few years of watching *Durham* in operation, I discussed this with the late Dr. Winfred Overholser, superintendent of St. Elizabeths, one of the foremost forensic psychiatrists of his day. He told me that the kind of information *Durham* was seeking would take from 50 to 100 hours of interviewing and investigation, and that the hospital simply could not provide those resources. I told him that psychiatrists should frankly explain on the witness stand how their opinions were thus affected by the limitations of time or facilities. This would cast no aspersion on their expertise. It was a far greater disservice to the legal process and the administration of justice for them to create the distorted impression that they had learned substantially all that could be known about someone on the basis of admittedly insufficient exploration and study. Rather than confront the court with these problems, psychiatrists swept them under the rug by rationalizing—as some have told me with commendable candor—that they were better able to balance the rights of the accused with the interest of society than either the court or the jury.

Moreover, psychiatrists ordinarily failed to disclose the differences of opinion, and the outright conflicts involved in psychiatric diagnosis by public hospital staffs. The jury was deprived of the staff opinions which disagreed with the official hospital recommendation. Attempts by my court to obtain records or tapes of just such clinical conferences have consistently been opposed and thwarted by the psychiatric staff at St. Elizabeths, the government's well-known mental hospital in Washington. (I might add that resistance to disclosure is not an uncommon phenomenon in Washington.)

After 15 years of such experience with *Durham,* my court last year in the *Brawner* case unanimously abandoned the *Durham* test. The *Brawner* decision essentially adopted the American Law Institute's proposed insanity test: "A person is not responsible for criminal conduct if at the time of such conduct as a result of mental disease or defect he lacks substantial capacity either to appreciate the wrongfulness of his conduct or to conform his conduct to the requirements of the law."

I instigated and favored the abandonment of *Durham* because, in practice, the *Durham* formulation had failed to elicit and provide through a disciplined investigation the necessary underlying information about the accused. The jury's function was once again usurped in rendering the ultimate moral judgment about blameworthiness.

While no phrase will magically solve the problem of expert dominance, my opinion in *Brawner* suggested the jury be instructed that a defendant is not responsible "if at the time of his unlawful conduct his mental or emotional processes or behavior controls were impaired to such an extent *that he cannot justly be held responsible.*" This approach envisions that the jury could be provided with a broad range of information about the accused from a variety of sources including but not necessarily limited to psychiatrists. The opportunity for other disciplines with special skills and knowledge in the field of human behavior to show the relevance of their data in the courtroom would not be precluded. Moreover, experts would be more likely to recognize that the question—whether it is *just* to blame the accused—involves moral and legal values beyond the parameters of their expertise. Even the promise of this approach would be broken unless means were provided for the defendant, who is virtually always indigent, to obtain and present the required broad spectrum of information.

The form of words we call the insanity defense is not crucial, but providing the jury with all arguably relevant information about the accused's freedom of choice is. As I said in *Brawner,* "while [we] generals are designing an inspiring new insignia for the standard, the battle is being lost in the trenches."

A major purpose of *Brawner* is to end the dominance by experts. But the *Brawner* formulation will not achieve this goal. It is designed to narrow the focus of the jury's inquiry rather than to expand it. Psychiatrists will continue to be the experts and they will take away the jury's function by presenting conclusory testimony.

Unfortunately, the purpose of *Durham* was thwarted by the professions' protective stance, and this attitude was unnecessary. In asking the profession to open up its opinions and decisions, the legal system was not out to "get" psychiatrists. It was asking only that when psychiatric expertise participates in public decisions it submit to the process by which the shortcomings of all opinion evidence are tested. Every doctor has a permanent emotional bias; he has an operational identification with an opinion which is used to support one side of the conflict; he has an inevitable identification with the accuracy of his own findings. Behavioral scientists are subject to the same prejudices as the rest of us, especially in respect to the criminal defendant, who often is not a person with whom one can easily empathize. These realities belie the myth that a medical expert can be removed from the legal adversary system.

I also saw organized psychiatry itself similarly respond in a protective, defensive stance to my opinions in *Jenkins,* which allowed psychologists to testify as experts on the insanity defense issue, and in *Rouse,* which focused on the right to treatment and to review of the adequacy of treatment for involuntarily committed patients.

In sum, it appeared that psychiatry was covering up more than the gaps in its knowledge. It was trying to conceal the conflicts between the imposition of treatment and the human and civil rights of patients. For the most part, professionals follow the line that there is *no* conflict, because *medical* decisions are, by definition, made in the best interests of the patient. If a doctor says the patient should be treated, or confined, or punished, it *must* be in his best interests because he *is* sick.

Such bootstrap assumptions are inevitably questioned whenever psychiatric decisions are exposed in the public sector, whether in the courtroom or in the community. Psychiatry uses the power of the state to confine people against their will. This necessarily introduces the potential for *misuse* of that power. It is a court's duty to scrutinize *all* governmental intrusions on freedom and liberty. The patient's interest in release, in less restrictive confinement, or in adequate treatment cannot be matters solely for "medical determination." Bringing these matters into court does not impose an artificial adversary posture between the patient and his keepers; it reflects the adversity which already exists.

Many of you probably sympathize with psychiatry's protective reaction to the challenge of the adversary process. Of course we all want to cover up our own limitations; it is tough to admit how much we do not know. But when I speak of the adversity which exists between psychiatrists and their so-called patients, I want to make it perfectly clear (to use a contemporary idiom) that at this point in time (to use yet another contemporary idiom) I am speaking particularly of institutional psychiatry.

Whenever psychiatrists enter the public sector to apply their knowledge at the request of public and social institutions—the military, or state hospitals, penal institutions, schools, to name only a few—they inevitably face conflicts between the therapeutic interests of their patients and the "institutional" interests of their employers. I also suspect that these conflicts are not resolved by their medical training or the Hippocratic oath. My eyes were really opened to this problem in discussions with personal friends and professional groups about the determinations they make; first, whether to commit a person to a hospital against his will; and, then, when to release him.

What I have heard over and over again is the frank admission that factors completely unrelated to a psychiatrist's medical expertise will form the basis for his decision to commit or release. At the Napa State Hospital in California a few years ago, the superintendent told me in a public meeting that the staff had "Sacramento looking over its shoulder" on all internal decisions. I learned in other contexts that psychiatric opinions are influenced by the public outcry for "law and order" and by personal fears for safety. In some hospitals shortages of bed space and manpower override medical considerations; in VA hospitals the need to fill empty beds produces the opposite result among voluntary patients. I have even been told by psychiatrists that they are justified in fudging their testimony on "dangerousness," where such a finding is required for commitment, if they are convinced that an individual is too sick to know that he needs help. It is not that psychiatric motives are venal, or that conflicting societal interests may dictate different results; we are used to that in the law. But it is frightening that psychiatrists do not bring these conflicts out into the open. Failure to do so fatally infects the decisional process. It takes serious legal and public challenges to bring to light the "hidden agendas" on which psychiatrists operate. For example, in most jurisdictions a finding of dangerousness is required in statutes governing civil commitment, conditional release, and sexual or other psychopathy. Efforts to have psychiatrists explain the basis for their recommendations have often met with extreme resistance. After attending a two-day conference on prediction of dangerousness a few years ago, I learned that the person who has committed the same crime 15 times is more likely to do it again than a person who is only a three-time, four-time, or eight-time repeater. I submit that for that insight you do not need to be an M.D. or have board certification.

Make no mistake, society was glad to throw this particular hot potato of predicting dangerousness into the collective psychiatric lap. But it is also distressing to think that many psychiatrists so readily accepted the delegation of such power without first determining whether their knowledge and skills were up to it, and that they are now trapped into pretending the potato is not very hot.

I have always believed that the process of testing expert opinion must start from within. The law even has a standard stock of tools to recommend. First, open up your decisions and make them public—if only to your colleagues. Record your staff conferences; keep your files. Initiate communication among yourselves by calling a *second* or a *third* decision-maker to advise you on crucial issues. When institutional interests come into play, take note of them— talk about them. Only then can you establish tentative criteria— if only for yourself—for resolving them. Like judicial precedents, these criteria will be flexible if they are out in the open. They will be useful if they are tested. They will approach wisdom if they are incorporated into the learning process. What I am suggesting is not novel. It is an accountability envisioned in peer review, which psychiatry, as well as medicine generally, should have begun long ago. Instead, it was left to Congress to do the job by enacting H.R. 1, which mandates peer review to begin January 1974 for all physicians, including psychiatrists, who receive funds under Medicare and Medicaid.

Some of my friends have heard me many times before urge psychiatrists to open up their locked doors. They call my preaching worthless because it is clear to them that psychiatry will *never* uncover its conflicts and will make me a scapegoat for suggesting it. Maybe they are right. I am certainly *less* optimistic about it—especially in view of my recent experience on a committee established by the Board of Trustees of the APA to explore conflicts in institutional psychiatry. After eight months of developing a research project, the committee was abolished under a barrage of ad hominem criticism.

The events over the eight-month period which led the APA to torpedo our project can be the topic of another speech. But I can tell you that by their action the APA had to disavow specifically the judgment of our committee members, including such establishment stalwarts as Harold Visotsky, the former director of mental health for the state of Illinois and present chairman of the Department of Psychiatry at Northwestern University; Ray Waggoner, a past president of the APA and retired chairman of the Department of Psychiatry at the University of Michigan; and John Visher, past speaker of the APA Assembly, and head of Mental Health Services for San Mateo County, California.

I believe that the psychiatric profession has much to gain from objective evaluation of its accomplishments. It is ironic—or it would be if it were not so tragic—that skepticism has grown to such proportions at a time when psychiatry has matured and has many achievements to be proud of: major breakthroughs in drug therapy; an increasing sophistication in examining behavior from a multidimensional or eclectic framework; and even an increasing sensitivity to the civil and human rights of patients, particularly among some of its youngest practitioners.

In my opinion, psychiatry has far more to gain than to lose if it responds positively to current challenges and undertakes a kind of *self*-analysis to ensure that its power rests on its expertise rather than its prestige. Therein lies the hope for psychiatry to develop more meaningful roles in society.

Bibliography

Bazelon, D. L.: Implementing the right to treatment. *University of Chicago Law Review,* Vol. 36, no. 4, Summer 1969.

——: The right to treatment: The court's role. *Hospital and Community Psychiatry,* Vol. 20, no. 5, May 1969.

Cross v. *Harris,* 418 F.2d 1095.

Durham v. *U.S.,* 214 F.2d 862.

Durham v. *U.S.,* 237 F.2d 760.

Jenkins v. *U.S.,* 307 F.2d 637.

McDonald v. *U.S.,* 312 F.2d 847.

Rouse v. *Cameron,* 373 F.2d 451.

U.S. v. *Alexander and Murdock,* 471 F.2d 923.

U.S. v. *Brawner,* 471 F.2d 1040.

U.S. v. *Eichberg,* 439 F.2d 620.

Washington v. *U.S.,* 419 F.2d 636.

13. The Role of Psychiatry in Society

Roy R. Grinker, Sr., M.D.

I T IS a great honor to participate in the 200th anniversary of Eastern State Hospital, once known as the Hospital for Lunatics and Idiots and, later, the Eastern Lunatic Asylum. These names do not indicate who were the lunatics and who were the idiots. Perhaps the latter term indicated the staff, identifiable by their possession of keys to the institution.

It should not be difficult for us to grasp the problems identified and the treatment methods used 200 years ago. Although I am not quite so old, I have witnessed during my own psychiatric career a repetition of the same problems and a recurring cycle of the same values and their approaches to etiology and treatment. Neuropathology (Grinker and Sahs 1966), at one time labeled Queen of the Sciences, dominated psychiatry under the later influence of Kraepelin, Nissl, and Alzheimer, and now again is asserting itself in the guise of psychopharmacology, leading back to secondary functional and/or morphological alterations. Reductionism, single causes, and linear chains from cause to effect are not dead issues. Moral treatment is now milieu therapy and plays a part in various kinds of community psychiatry.

Despite the heavy burden of many old and primitive approaches there is much that is new and, I hope, valuable for the future. But I shall not attempt to predict the future of psychiatry since I possess only a fractional knowledge of the past and focal interest in the present. We can predict the future with any assurance only in terms of present societies: *that it be more so and better than!* There is, however, a new "science" called futurology that deals less with prediction and more with generalities that allow for uncertainties and the unpredictable (Marojama 1972). Goal-generating thinking or what I have called goal-changing processes are stimulated or catalyzed by challenges. Freedom for such creativity is favored by education in transepistemological processes.

All sciences, including their primitive precursor, mythology

(Frazer 1932), are closely involved, either directly or indirectly, in their contemporary social matrix. Psychiatry is in part a social science since man is a social animal, for good or ill, and his individuality is only approximate, not ultimate. Society demands, requests, condones and condemns some forms of psychiatry just as it deals with other intellectual trends in its component members or groups. In this sense psychiatry is *in* society. In another sense psychiatry and society are two systems closely related to one another by transactions across their interface. The interface between society and medicine, including psychiatry, is stated clearly by Charles Johnson (Grinker 1953*a*): "Social sciences furnish foundations which enable psychiatry to link medicine with social situations within the broad control of culture." To understand this relationship one has to designate those parts of society with which psychiatry exchanges information. These include the family, the neighborhood and other geographical partitions, the school, police, church, work, etc.

Until humans accept the Mankind concept with its overarching, all-embracing recognition of a conspecics, society as a global concept has little practical or operational value. On the other hand, one of psychiatry's major problems is its vagueness, diffusion, and confusion of terms. The field's vocabulary is neither consensual within itself or with bordering systems, and we are correctly accused of speaking and writing in jargon. Even within the field, terms are not adequately defined in theory or operations. Think of the many words borrowed from physics such as psychic *energy*, or quantitative statements such as *cathexis* or *neutralization of aggressive energy.*

Joseph Fletcher (1972) defines positive human criteria as a minimal intelligence, self-consciousness, self-control, a sense of time, a sense of the future and the past, concern for others, communications with others, control of existence, curiosity, change and changeability, and balance of rationality and feeling. He states that good answers to the question of the nature of man "are more apt to be found inductively and empirically from medical science and the clinicians than by the necessarily syllogistic reasoning of the humanities."

Obviously within these simple, easily understandable statements there are no connotations of "positive mental health" (Yahoda 1958). However, we cannot avoid discussing the heavily value-laden and biased concepts of health, normality, and illness in considering psychiatry and society. Strupp (Strupp 1972) defines health and illness as follows: "The normal individual has 'come to terms' with the problem of social illness and has succeeded in modulating it; the neurotic continues to make an issue of it; and the psychopath has largely turned his back on it." Whitehorn and Betz (1957) state that the healthy person loves well, plays well, and expects well.

Society determines what mental health is for its population (Grinker 1962). As Ira in Mell's cartoon said in answer to his teacher's question, "Ira, don't you want to be known as a normal, average, American boy?": "No, I want to be like all the others." Health is a value system dependent on the place, time, and population. Each set of conditions imposes a threshold beyond which deviance becomes intolerable and is termed illness. Anselm Strauss (Strauss et al. 1964) has stated: "We need much more sophistication about normality—a sociological range and differentiation of normal behavior now almost altogether missing in the psychiatrist's thinking."

Society lays down not only standards for health and for the acceptance of the secondary role of illness, but also the means by which coping mechanisms may be used in the stresses of development, which seem to be phase-specific, and in the threatening events and crises in our turbulent lives. "Normality and illness are only polarities of a wide range of integrations. . . . When strained, the organismic systems respond according to the processes by which the many subvariances have become integrated. . . . thus, the degree of health and illness in the stress responses reveals the quality and quantity of integration" (Grinker 1967a).

Having indicated so far the close relationship between psychiatry and society, I shall now attempt to define not "psychiatry" but the *multiple* "psychiatries" as they have evolved and as they exist today. The lay public has come to think of psychiatrists as doctors practicing a branch of medicine. This indeed they do, although after medical school and graduate training most of them promptly forget all they have learned about the body, refusing to touch it as if it were abhorrent.

For the socioeconomically higher classes a psychiatrist uses words or interpretations almost exclusively, and is called a *psychotherapist*. Psychotherapy is old. Hippocrates relied on expectations that the baths, rest, beautiful environment, and favorable climate at his hospital would cure many. The witch doctors of Africa still, after years of training, use impressive surroundings, strange instruments, ununderstandable words, and high fees to achieve good results. Indeed, the nonspecific elements of all therapies seem to be the crucial factors of recovery. Each school of therapy uses its own methods for everything. Who directs the patient to which, and why? It is indeed true that psychotherapy, dynamic or otherwise, is a dominant treatment modality in psychiatric practice, but it has been reinforced by acceptance and demands from a segment of society. More than that, psychiatrists have influenced social-work therapists, clinical psychologists, and, latterly, nurses to conduct individual, group, and family psychotherapy.

A second group of psychiatrists are called *somatotherapists* because they adhere strictly to the medical model, utilizing electric shock whenever possible and a wide range of drugs. These include the antischizophrenic and antidepressive drugs as well as lithium for manic attacks, singly or in combination. True, they say they also do psychotherapy, but a few kind words and greetings can hardly deserve such a term. On the other hand, psychotherapists are increasingly willing to use drugs as adjuncts and facilitators for their own brand of therapy. This was not always so, because when the phenothiazines first appeared, Sabshin and Ramot (1956) reported that our psychotherapists were reluctant to use drugs, or used them in insufficient doses. The entire social field composed of doctors and nurses was biased against the use of drugs, and the results were less positive than in other methods during the 1950s. Now, with a strongly positive bias, the social field reinforces the value of medication to the extent that it has become more difficult to evaluate the effect of any form of treatment by itself.

Another evidence of interaction between society and psychiatric therapists is the treatment of socioeconomically low patients in crisis. Many psychiatrists have the idea that such patients are not suitable for psychotherapy, but this is not true although many such patients do consider psychiatrists as doctors, demand medication at once, and hurry to leave the hospital to return to the job and/or home. Once they go it is extremely difficult to persuade them to continue treatment on an outpatient basis.

A third group of psychiatrists may be called *sociotherapists.*

These emphasize milieu therapy in the hospital, and group or family therapy for both in- and outpatients. They veer away from the medical model more than the others (although not entirely, as Albee [1971] recommends), not only in their treatment modality but in their denigration of diagnostic terms and specific therapies. Instead, they repudiate the concept of illness, substituting for it "disturbances resulting from problems in living." Society has in part accepted this distinction and has become enamored with so-called encounter groups to the dismay of many of us.

An altogether different social form of therapy, based on the philosophy of Kierkegaard, is conducted by the existentialists. Beck (1972) contrasted the patriarch Abraham, who disobeyed the ethics of the pagan god by refusing to kill his son and thereby created a new ethic, with Kierkegaard, who continually vacillated between resignation and conformity, and self-assertion and action. To quote Beck: "Either, or. In confusion and disorganization they have opted for the pleasure principle, which still leaves them in turbulent imbalance."

The existential psychiatrist attempts to help patients who are afraid of not being free to find themselves unless they dichotomize themselves and the socioeconomic world to which they are bound on this earth. But these people cannot leave by means of hallucinatory drugs or by living in isolated communes. They can be free selves only as part of the society in which they live.

The three models that have been described correspond to the definition of psychiatry as a medical specialty devoted to the diagnosis and treatment of mental illness. The sharpness of the separation among them is blurring more and more. But diagnostic criteria and, for that matter, interest in diagnosis are in a total mess, and so therapy in psychiatry cannot be considered as even an applied science. Thus in a psychology conference on graduate education in the 1940s it was said that psychotherapy is an undefined technic applied to unspecified problems with unpredictable results. Yet rigorous training in this technic is recommended.

What then is the science of psychiatry, if there is such a field? How is it different from the delivery of services for which there is little enquiry or evaluation? Society is interested in services and often demands instant results, but how do we learn more about human problems in order to satisfy the needs and demands of society? I quote from the cogent essay of my colleague Daniel X. Freedman:

Such a society, especially a technological society, would come to value science as a social system through which the understanding of nature and human nature is advanced. They would, on reflection, appreciate that this happens through a mode of activities that conserves, adjudicates, accumulates and transforms knowledge, a mode that transcends the ability of single individuals as well as generations. The business of doing this involves investigators, doers and appliers. It involves scholars who look back for perspective and critical teachers who, comprehending the contingent status of knowledge, equip the young for the unknown future. Such a system incidentally goes against our intrinsic megalomanic and wishful trends. It requires some valuing of objectivity and the ability to see the unwanted, to be jolted from custom and belief, to tolerate ambiguity and delay of gratification in pursuit of the future, and to enjoy such discipline and insecurity for the intellectual payoff and, once in a while, for the actual practical gain. Such values conserve knowledge but they also underwrite, expect and anticipate change. Such values challenge our imperfections while perfecting our mastery of them (Freedman 1972).

In his famous book *The Golden Bough,* James Frazer (1932) described the common primitive roots of science and magic, both of which follow general rules. Magic developed into religion with belief in powers higher than man. These must be propitiated in true faith, whether they be gods or God, drugs, leaders of the various social systems now springing up anew as multiple aberrant communes or as singularly led encounter groups, or even existential faith in self. Psychiatry still seems magical to some, but society's faith in psychiatry's powers has waned and in many places turned to overt or covert contempt. In an era of anti-intellectualism, psychiatry has in some degree joined the general return to mysticism, for man fails without faith or hope of some kind. Faith in research is too abstract and uncertain to be maintained.

This mysticism has taken two general forms. One is the emphasis on a new humanism, even a mutation (Gerber 1972) of consciousness to an integration of a "perspective world." The other is a mystical overevaluation of a human figure in which he is made into a faultless God as Eissler made Freud (Eissler 1965).

Some time in the latter part of the 1950s, research and clinical psychiatrists became self-conscious when they suddenly discovered that psychiatry was an integral part of the vast field of behavioral sciences (Luszki 1958). Their focus could no longer scotomatize larger areas of behavior such as the biological, psychological, social, or economic. Ideas of unified or systems theory seem to furnish answers in their concepts of openness, communications, transactions, homeostasis, and isomorphism. Thus clinical psychiatry began to participate in social action under increased political freedom and at the same time research psychiatry absorbed field theories.

Many years of resistance against a general theory of mental health and illness were influenced by the fact that psychiatry for so long had been dominated by psychoanalysis, which had its own umbrella called metapsychology. When scientific or research psychiatry became part of the behavioral sciences a general theory was needed to counteract the parochialism of its contributory sciences. Yet few authors were actually doing research; they philosophized, and many resolved dilemmas prematurely by mathematical equations in a language poorly understood by the empirical investigator.

Gradually, more and more psychiatrists became interested, and organized their own special groups, hoping to communicate in a common language that was consonant and not disjunctive with their own biological, psychological, and social models. They were tired of senseless controversy about who knows *the* cause of health and illness; they became convinced of multicausality and reciprocal relations rather than linearity of cause and effect. As a result the probabilities of a systems approach were enhanced. This is not to assume that any scientist could cover the entire field of the behavioral sciences; but he could feel more comfortable knowing where he was instead of endlessly riding around in search of boundaries.

Psychiatrists began to recognize that systems and subsystems constituting hierarchies, and bounded by permeable borders that encased reverberating transactions, had structure-functions and integrative processes. But, more than that, they realized that a system functions in relation to other systems. In fact, the proof or validation of a system's functions cannot come from within but depends on its "purpose" in relation to another system. This respectable teleology lends meaning to human research which is, admittedly or not, the goal of science rather than a game that we enjoy playing.

Systems approach to the social sciences accentuates human symbolic functions that are the essence of humanity in the individual, in the group, or in society. It is deviation in development, disturbance in integration, and failure to react conservatively to disturbing human or inanimate stimuli from the environment that constitute the essence of disease. When we think of society and psychiatry as science in modern terms of systems it is possible to think of psychiatry as part of a social system composed of many other parts. Thus the larger social system may condone, condemn, or support change, recognizing research as fulfillment of the need to search, to change our notion of man, and to enhance the quality of living.

A more productive way of looking at psychiatry as a system (Grinker 1966) in order to preclude reductionism and/or humanness as dichotomies, is to represent society, within the sciences of sociology and anthropology, as part of the psychiatric system. We conceive of psychiatry as a biopsychosocial system which (Grinker 1973) attempts to synthesize behavioral sciences into a unified theory of human behavior. I need not repeat the biological and psychological components for this audience or within the confines of my subject. What is important is the fact that social and personality components are interdependent and that they interpenetrate. All parts constitute an organization that is controlled and regulated by the unifying principle of survival or homeostasis; this encompasses stability, growth, evolution, social organization, increasing complexity, and optimum variability. Emerson (1954) states that the scientific principle of homeostasis assists in the resolution of many controversies and dilemmas. It is both a mechanism and a trend of life processes. It indicates the gaps in our knowledge and understanding, and it directs future investigations.

We are becoming increasingly aware of the reciprocal relationship among personality characteristics that under certain conditions predispose an individual to the full-blown disorder, disease, or deviance (whichever term is preferred). This reciprocal movement is clear in depressive (Grinker et al. 1961), borderline (Grinker, Weble, and Drye 1968), and schizophrenic (Grinker 1969) patients. Movement from disease state back to character traits is the most that can be hoped for from any therapy.

Our concepts of the multiple causes of emotional and cognitive disturbances and their treatment are certainly dependent on our view as observers of the transactions among social and cultural processes and those of the personality. Granted the innate biological basis of some diseases, are subsequent personality deviances due to difficult or traumatic experiences in early family life? How much do conflicts in society contribute to psychological malfunctioning? We have begun to realize that each phase of childhood, adolescence, young adulthood, adulthood, and aging, has its own conflicts, predispositions, susceptibilities, forms of deviance, and applicable therapies. Nor is society a uniform phenomenon. Ours is not a unitary society as the mythology of the melting pot described it. It is, indeed, a pluralistic society composed of various ethnic and socioeconomic groups with different colors of people. Our states and regions are still differentiated by their geography, resources, and industries. Our so-called two-party political system reveals itself as an aggregate of coalitions held together by the character or schemes of their leaders. Just as we cannot speak of *a psychiatry* we cannot speak of *a society*. A person is exposed to the society and culture of the place in which he is born and where he subsequently lives; of the schools he attends and the milieu in which he works. They make demands upon him to adapt, and they differ significantly from place to place within our country. The move from one place to another, even over so short a distance as that from a city to its suburbs, or the retreat from a neighborhood through which a thruway is working its destructive course, requires new and different forms of coping.

Thus we have systems in process in constant movement, with individuals growing, maturing, developing into different phases of the life cycle, and society changing with incredible speed because of technological discoveries. A one-to-one relationship, a matching between personality or psychopathy and sociocultural factors, is thus very difficult. This has always been so although psychiatrists have ignored the rapidly shifting internal and external factors involved in psychiatry. Recognition now results in less certainty, albeit greater sophistication in research, as controlling for many variables has become more difficult.

So far we have discussed psychiatry and society as systems with their own parts and regulatory functions, interpenetrating so that one can become part of the other, and vice versa—or so they may transact as separate systems. But society has little regard for the conceptual and abstract, or little investment in its future. Immediate action is demanded. Drugs appropriate for specific conditions are almost universally ingested in order to make the taker "feel better." Behavioral therapy short-cuts insight, and freedom is sacrificed so that people may be shaped into desirable molds. The social fickleness of American society is exemplified in its rapid shift of bandwagons (Grinker 1964), and psychiatry likewise "rides madly in all directions."

We are still being influenced by the attitudes of big-business government. It was expressed by Charles Wilson of General Motors, who said that "basic research" is the term used when you do not know what you are doing. So we are asked to do target research or research of relevance. But who knows what is relevant and where the target is? Nobelist Szent-Györgyi tells the story of how his faked projects were supported and his realistic projects rejected by the "popes of the field."

Concern now seems to be focused on the so-called community psychiatry, much of which is good but much pure fantasy. Community mental health centers are not instruments of primary prevention. Few know what prevention means, and no one knows how to effect it. The centers are distribution areas, not instruments of social change, and psychiatrists are not social engineers. Neither are they politicians able to lobby well for their own purposes, nor do they do well with the local community's board of directors. Statements of opinion about social issues should be made by psychiatrists only as citizens. Official and professional opinions are only for the purpose of advising on procedures to further mental health and to point out what actions are detrimental.

We have been duped by our own professional bureaucrats who have assumed a political role as advisers to the various governmental agencies. They assume that they speak for the workers in the field. Promises of prevention have been made for as long as I remember. The possibility of curing everybody by anything seems to be accepted by the public each time a new name is invented. The profession has been split by bureaucrats belaboring a "private sector" when, indeed, most practitioners hold part-time jobs and most psychiatrists working in public hospitals do part-time practice.

Before World War II we thought psychiatry was enjoying a breakthrough into the causes of those physical ailments called psychosomatic. Specificity of emotions and characterological cliches was expected to pinpoint foci for therapeutic attack. Unfortunately, our war experiences (Grinker and Spiegel 1945) and subsequent postwar studies revealed that specificity was not on the causal side of the chain but on the response side. Thus research into the mind-body (stress-response) must move toward the biogenetic and early experiences which form the basis of specific responses to meaningful stress (Grinker 1953b).

There are some indications that despite our lack of progress we are learning how to ask the right questions. In a recent symposium on schizophrenia Kety (1972) asked 17 questions. In 1969 I asked 12 questions which overlap Kety's but are more oriented toward a systems approach (Grinker 1967b).

We do have grave responsibilities toward society, as does all of medicine. These transcend our specific professionalism, which is dedicated to preserving and improving human life. Once we tamper with everyone's right to live, no matter what the cost, we sacrifice our democratic way of life and eventually degenerate into a genocidal culture. Yet there are ethical problems raised by the Hastings Institute; these include death and dying, behavioral control, population policy, and genetic counseling. There is a more pressing ethical issue for psychiatrists than keeping the mentally retarded and the hopelessly senile alive. With increasing confidence that there is a biological basis to the development of the schizophrenic system we should be aware that we are increasing the genetic pool by the use of antischizophrenic drugs, the discharge of patients from "warehouses," and the facilitating of marriage and childbearing among the schizophrenic population.

As I said at the beginning of this presentation, I cannot predict the future of psychiatry. I am not sanguine about the future, not only because we are in an era of anti-intellectualism with anti-psychiatric attitudes but also because I see the profession itself downgraded by destructive and splintering behavior within its own ranks.

A recent Ciba Foundation Conference (Ciba Foundation Symposium 1972), although without any reference to psychiatry and without a single psychiatric participant, discussed the current anti-scientific movement that blames scientists for ruining the golden age of mankind. Science is tolerated today only if it is socially relevant, and scientists are criticized for a lack of social responsibility and a lack of values. There is a movement for evaluation and control of science for its relevancy. Science is considered to be in conflict with humanism, ignoring individuality, imagination, and quality. A plea is being made for a framework of institutional policy-making in the interest of the nonscientific majority.

Lord Robert Hargreaves is quoted as saying that rats leave a sinking ship but that it is unusual for rats to sink the ship. Yet this is just what is being done by our publicity-seeking brethren who speak authoritatively on any subject. Some promise what they cannot achieve. Statistics are garbled by the "revolving door" results of tranquilizing all patients without dealing with their basic problems. The chairmen of departments of psychiatry travel more than they work at their tasks at home. We must take a share of the blame for the denigration of our specialty by society.

As some schizophrenic patients have said to me, "We are the sane—you are the crazy ones." Maybe so! Nevertheless, when we look at the scoreboard of the last 200 years, even though time is running short, we still have the opportunity to combat those who would hold us back. We should be able to influence society to cooperate rather than fight us as we attempt to effect a better way of life and to neutralize the destructive processes that impinge on all mankind.

Bibliography

Albee, G.: Emerging concepts of mental illness and models of treatment: The psychologist's point of view. *American Journal of Psychiatry* 125:869–76, 1969. Also in *Professional Psychology* 2:128–45, 1971.

Beck, S. J.: Abraham and Kierkegaard: Either, Or. *Yale Review of Biology and Medicine* 62:54–75, 1972.

Ciba Foundation Symposium: *Civilization and Science in Conflict or Collaboration.* North Holland: Elsevier-Excerpta Medica, 1972.

Eissler, K. R.: *Medical Orthodoxy and the Future of Psychoanalysis.* New York: International Universities Press, 1965.

Emerson, A. E.: Dynamic homeostasis: A unifying principle in organic, social and ethical evolution. *Scientific Monthly* 78:67–85, 1954.

Fletcher, J.: *Hastings Center Report,* Vol. 2, November 1972.

Frazer, J. G.: The Golden Bough: A Study in Magic and Religion. 3d ed. New York: Macmillan, 1932, I:220–43.

Freedman, D. X.: Can we put research to work? *Highlights of the 17th Annual Conference of VA Cooperative Studies in Mental Health and the Behavioral Sciences, St. Louis, Mo., March, 1972.*

Gerber, J.: The foundations of the perspective world. Trans. Lerdecker, K. F. *Main Currents in Modern Thought* 29:80–88, 1972.

Grinker, R. R., Sr. (ed.) : *Midcentury Psychiatry*. Springfield, Ill.: Charles C. Thomas, 1953*a*.

———: *Psychosomatic Research*. New York: Norton, 1953*b*.

———: Mentally healthy young males (homoclites) : *Archives of General Psychiatry* 6:404–53, 1962.

———: Psychiatry rides madly in all directions. *Archives of General Psychiatry* 10:228, 1964.

———: "Open-system" psychiatry. *American Journal of Psychoanalysis* 26:115–28, 1966.

———: Normality viewed as a system. *Archives of General Psychiatry* 17:320–24, 1967*a*.

——— (ed.) : *Toward a Unified Theory of Human Behavior*. 2d ed. New York: Basic Books, 1967*b*.

———: An essay on schizophrenia and science. *Archives of General Psychiatry* 20:1–24, 1969.

———: The relevance of general systems theory to psychiatry. In *American Handbook of Psychiatry*. Arieti, S. (ed.). Vol. 6, Hamburg and Brody (eds.). New York, Basic Books, 1973.

———, and Spiegel, J.: *Men under Stress*. Philadelphia: Blakiston, 1945.

———, Miller, J., Sabshin, M., and Nunnally, J. C.: *The Phenomena of Depression*. New York: Hoeber, 1961.

———, and Sahs, A.: *Neurology*. 6th ed. Springfield, Ill.: Charles C. Thomas, 1966.

———, Weble, R., and Drye, R. C.: *The Borderline Syndrome*. New York: Basic Books, 1968.

Kety, S., and Matthysse, S. (eds.) .: Prospects for research on schizophrenia. *Neurosciences Research Program Bulletin*, Vol. 10, no. 4, November 1972.

Luszki, M. D. (ed.) : *Interdisciplinary Team Research*. New York: New York University Press, 1958.

Marojama, M.: Toward human futuristics. *General Systems Theory* 17:3–15, 1972.

Sabshin, M., and Ramot, J.: Psychotherapeutic evaluation and the psychiatric setting. *AMA Archives of Neurology and Psychiatry* 75:362, 1956.

Strauss, A., Schatzman, L., Bucher, R., Ehrlich, D., and Sabshin, M.: *Psychiatric Ideologies and Institutions*. New York: Free Press of Glencoe, 1964.

Strupp, H. H.: On the technic of psychotherapy. *Archives of General Psychiatry* 26:270–78, 1972.

Whitehorn, J. C., and Betz, B. J.: A comparison of psychotherapeutic relationship between physicians and schizophrenic patients. *American Journal of Psychiatry* 113:901–10, 1957.

Yahoda, N.: *Current Concepts of Positive Mental Health*. New York: Basic Books, 1958.

Discussion

DR. HAWKINS: I will start by asking if any one of the speakers wishes to amplify his remarks or address questions or comments to any of the other speakers. I know there are some questions from the audience, and Dr. Sabshin would like to make some comments.

DR. SABSHIN: It has been a fascinating series of papers. I will make a few brief comments and put a question or two to some of the speakers. Professor Rosenberg described a variety of structural problems besetting psychiatry. I believe he separates psychiatry from the rest of medicine to a degree that goes a step or two beyond what I would endorse. I am currently an acting dean, and in that sense I have an enormous opportunity for sociological fieldwork with other medical disciplines. I would say that if you analyze these disciplines carefully, some of the problems that he described as besetting psychiatry do indeed exist in them too. If you watch what is happening in pathology and note the struggles between clinical pathologists and experimental pathologists, and the struggles about teaching versus basic research, you see that the problems are there as well. If you look at the role of family practice as an emerging specialty and its position in university departments, you see that many of the same social forces as those troubling psychiatrists play a role in producing problems in that field also. You can see a considerable degree of marginality in the area of public health and preventive medicine. So I raise this question: I do not deny that psychiatry has many marginal elements, but has the structural analysis of other specialties been so superficial as to exaggerate the differences?

One other question for Professor Rosenberg is this: When he raised questions about the difficulty in evaluating, measuring, or quantifying the role of nonpsychiatrists in psychological medicine, does not the same problem pertain to evaluating the work of psychiatrists themselves? I submit that there are some developments that may improve at least our evaluation of educational programs. So I think the difficulties and problems are somewhat exaggerated by the way he described the issue, although, in general, I agree with many of his points.

The brilliantly defended plea of Professor Schwartz poses a problem for me; let me try to convey it to you. I do not agree that de-humanization is necessarily spreading in our society in this latter part of the 20th century. I think that if we looked over the history of past centuries we would see that de-humanization has been the experience of most of the people of the world in most societies. Is the key to our present acute awareness of de-humanization the fact that it has begun to affect the upper middle classes, the intellectual world, so that we are more affected ourselves? I ask if that may not be true. What is the evidence that for most people in the world de-humanization is really more marked now? If it is, it affects greater numbers of people and reaches the class that we represent. Is there a danger that in coping with this problem we may find a very interesting and perhaps paradoxical rationalization for our work in individual psychotherapy—that at least we are trying to provide some more humanizing experiences for patients able to afford our services—while we still avoid trying to do anything comparable for the masses? If, on the other hand, Professor Schwartz is really interested in seeing that we become change agents and express these value systems, I would submit that he comes into conflict with one of Dr. Grinker's cautions. Is our role really one of becoming agents of specific change or one of elucidating data or attempting to advise other decision-makers? And if we assume the role of change agents, where do we stop?

To Judge Bazelon I would say simply that some people promised you a rose garden; you expected less, but you got even less than you expected. Certainly many people made those kinds of promissory statements, but he has been working in an arena that exposes all our weaknesses and all our lack of knowledge; and the conceptual difficulties that Dr. Grinker recognizes in the terminology used to describe health and illness are, in my judgment, underlying problems in dealing with the courtroom situation. We can be more reliable when we talk about gross abnormalities, and indeed we can find some consensus in the *McNaughten* decision. But in the absence of the kind of data that are really convincing to us—that is, to those of us who ponder this subject and acknowledge the limitations—I think the facts are that the distinctions between health and illness, and the causation of certain behaviors, are an Achilles' heel for us in many ways. The courtroom situation exposes our weaknesses and our heterogeneity beyond belief. I think there is some opportunity for dialogue about this. I have told Judge Bazelon this, so it is not being said behind his back, but I think his experience of 24 years can serve as a grim reminder of some of the things that we do not know and that we should acknowledge that we do not know.

As for Dr. Grinker, I think no one in psychiatry in this century has done more to try to develop a new kind of synthesis than he has through the general systems theory that he proposed; but he is able at this time to acknowledge the weaknesses in that attempt. I would call your attention to how relevant his comments are for discussion about *Durham,* and for questions about health and morality, but how his questions about the approach to humanization can also be distorted into a kind of new anti-intellectualism and a force for mysticism. There is a curious bypath in that area, one that in many ways the group therapist, encounter groups, and the existentialist have indeed taken. They espouse humanization, but to what extent are they really providing a kind of safety valve for certain people who could not get into the human dimension in their families or in some other social institution?

DR. ROSENBERG: I do not see a real need for discussion because I think the differences we have are relatively trivial. I was not speaking at that point from a prepared speech, but I recall saying that all areas of applied science suffer from the same kinds of problems in communication and structure, and, although it may be that psychiatry is peculiar in some ways, every other field is peculiar in its own way too. I think one might make the case that this failure to develop cultural artifacts does make psychiatry a little different. I think we have to discuss that, but I am glad that he agrees with my general point.

DR. SCHWARTZ: There are a number of things I would like to say. Let me start with Dr. Sabshin's last statement about the conception of humanization's moving, at least in some areas, toward mysticism. I am not afraid of mysticism. Evidently if you are a scientist you are not supposed to be mystical. I think I can contain both points of view in my personality; at least I try to, and it does not make me ill. The second point that I would make is that humanization does not necessarily move in that direction. I could think of its being very concrete, and that is what I was trying to specify when I gave you my definition, that what it means to humanize another person in a concrete, specific way is to treat him as an end in himself. But even if humanization does move in the direction of mysticism, perhaps we are depriving ourselves of something by not permitting ourselves to experience the mystical as well as the scientific. If I remember correctly, there are some great physicists now who are coming to that point of view—that there is no conflict between being a great scientist and also having a mystical sense of the universe.

The second question was: Where do you stop? I do not know where you stop. I ask: Where do you begin? Before you wonder where you are going to stop you had better start at the beginning; otherwise that question does not make sense. If you agree with my analysis that there is this very intimate, intricate relationship between the nature of our institutions and the nature of our individual pathology, and if you psychiatrists are the agents for doing something about this pathology, then I do not see how you can ignore the institutional sources of the pathology. Now you can play the role of adviser, which you have done (although nothing much happens as a result), and you can try to get more actively involved. I am not trying to tell you what to do, but it seems to me that you might experiment to try to get a little closer toward that activist role.

Now perhaps all our conceptions about its being unprofessional to be activist might be broken down a little bit. We can ask ourselves the question: Can you be a professional and at the same time take a value-committed stance? I say I think you can. I think you take a value stance anyway, whether you make it explicit or not. I tried to indicate in my talk that a value stance is either in support of what already is or actively opposed to what already is, particularly in respect to humanization and de-humanization. This, then, leads to the last point, the point of penetration. That is why I emphasized specifically that psychiatry is, presumably at least, dedicated to the humanizing principle in its ideology. It seems to me that the critical point of penetration is where you can try to do something about institutions.

Now the question Dr. Sabshin raised as to whether humanization is increasing or decreasing is an impossible question to answer. I do not know whether it is increasing or decreasing; my guess would be that in many ways it is increasing and in some ways it is decreasing. Psychiatry, in its emphasis on the individual, helps to decrease de-humanization, but technology, science, and mass society help to increase it. I would not know how to weigh one against the other—that is not the point. The fact is that de-humanization is pervasive, powerful, inescapable—and in many ways unrecognized. I think psychiatry can have a critical role to play in bringing out the subtle as well as the overt ways in which de-humanization works in our society and how it interweaves with a kind of emotional disturbance that gets labeled as neurosis or psychosis or whatever.

DR. HAWKINS: One of the questions that came from the audience is along the lines we have just been considering. This is addressed to Dr. Schwartz and the panel: What do you see as the possible positive and/or negative effects on our profession when psychiatrists in their role as psychiatrists and not in their role as private citizens take partisan political positions and become actively involved in social change?

DR. GRINKER: I think I would like to emphasize again that we have no business except to give to the agencies concerned with making rules and regulations, laws and the like, the information we acquire through the study of healthy and sick people. I will give you an example. I interviewed for a questionnaire a large number of healthy young males, calling them homoclites in order to avoid the value system implied in the words *normal* and *healthy*. They all went to George Williams College; they all had an almost straight-line kind of development, early involvement in work, religion, YMCA experiences, and so on; and they all went to this YMCA college to prepare themselves to be settlement house leaders, group leaders, or something similar. This is all a part of their cultural social life, in almost a straight line. Then along came a new president, a George Williams graduate who had taken his Ph.D. degree in sociology somewhere else. He decided this school was too small and too restricted. The young men who went there were called "muscular Christians" by University of Chicago students. They were called "the upright young men" because they wanted to do good for other people and did not care about making large incomes. The new president said, "We've got to move." So he asked me what would happen if the school moved. I said, "You will have students who will be the same kind of neurotic and psychotic students that the University of Chicago has." He said, "Well, we've got to move anyway."

So when I went there just about six months ago to give a talk I noticed that they had student counselors. They had a psychologist to help students in trouble, and they had a regular run of college student troubles. So I had done my best to advise them against de-humanizing a small, lovely college, but what good did it do? Nothing! I cannot pass a law saying you cannot move a small college into university status. I mind my own business and tell when they ask (or give advice even when I am not asked) about what I see are the factors involved that will cause illness and those that will maintain health. When I was in a fascist society during the war—that is, in the army—I did have one social function. I could reclassify the soldier. I could say, "You are not fit for this job; you are not fit to be here." But I cannot do that in a democracy.

DR. SCHWARTZ: I hope I am not leaving the impression that I want the psychiatrist to become supreme authority in our society. That is far from my intention. What I am trying to ask is, Are there any places in the arena where you can make the kinds of interventions that would make a difference? Can you orient your patients to look upon their pathology as something that not only represents an intrapsychic or intrafamilial difficulty but is also related to society as a whole? Can you do something about their immediate social environment?

Once you get a perspective of focusing on the social environment or on the social system or on whatever institution you are involved in, there are multitudinous ways to act. You may start to wonder what kinds of intervention you want to make to alter the system. I do not see how in the world we are ever going to deal with this problem of emotional disturbance in our society if the institutions which are so powerful and dominant continue to turn out emotionally disturbed persons.

Every once in a while I read a report from Detroit on how many people are breaking down on the production line in the automobile factories, and everybody seems to believe their breakdown is a direct consequence of the horrible conditions under which they work. That is a very simple example of where an institutional process is almost immediately productive of severe emotional disturbance. Now I do not believe that a psychiatrist can go in there and tell Henry Ford to stop his production line. But there are ways in which you can make inroads, direct or indirect, that you have not thought about before. All that I am asking for is some kind of imaginative exploration of how to move into the arena a little more actively. I do not expect you to be able to take over or to give orders to anybody to change things.

DR. HAWKINS: I would like to return to one of Dr. Sabshin's questions. Do we in fact clearly have the data on which to base the notion that we should make a major move in this direction? Certainly we talk about things like the assembly line as being conducive to emotional distress, but how much do we *know* about it? Are you not perhaps leading us again into the trap of trying to push prematurely for certain aims? In light of Judge Bazelon's comment that he hoped that getting psychiatrists into the courtroom would irrigate the wasteland—as if simply bringing out in the courtroom some of the problems that we work with and face all the time would lead to any further understanding—it seems to me that is not the way to get further understanding. I wonder whether one really has data to go on, and whether we may not be trapped somewhat in our own social system. For example, as we hear a bit from the Chinese now one begins to feel that there may be a great deal wrong with the emphasis on the individual in Western society and with our competitive struggles, and that perhaps we ought to be a bit more content to occupy our places in society without always struggling for individualism. Of course, this may not be quite what you are getting at when you speak of humanization, but maybe you would comment on this possibility.

DR. SCHWARTZ: My comment is simply this: Do you have the data to support your belief that the individual disturbances you see in your patients are caused by biochemical deviance or by family and mother-child relationships? You are making assumptions, some adopting one set of assumptions more ardently than another. It seems to me that it is impossible to get the kind of conclusive data that one would want, to enter the arena we are talking about, and that you are persuaded mostly by your frame of reference and your predispositions. I will admit to my own. And I think that everyone should ask himself this question.

DR. HAWKINS: To that I would only say that, poor as our data are in all areas that relate to our profession, I do think we have somewhat more understanding and somewhat more reliable data about some of the biological issues—and perhaps in some of the issues concerned with individual psychological development. However, I certainly do not want to take the point of view that social forces are not of great importance. I think our being able to contribute is more a matter of timing. I think many of us are sensitive to premature statements about what we can or cannot do because we have been burned before.

DR. ROSENBERG: There is no need to phrase this debate in terms of either/or. It is a question of balancing the total intellectual input. I think that most of us will agree that there has been comparatively little emphasis generally throughout the profession on studying the relationship between social structure and social role, and on possible effects of their impingement on the individual's development. I am thinking of certain of the social issues raised over the past few years. The most conspicuous, perhaps, is the so-called women's liberation movement, which concerns 51 percent of the population. I think that whether or not the issues as formulated now are sound, it has brought up a variable that has not had sufficient study, and I think your discipline is in a funny position when your research concerns are defined for you by what emerges from social ferment and social change. I think there are very few people in this room who would not be influenced, to some extent at least, by this movement when they see a female patient or when they are thinking about research that might be done in their own institution.

DR. HAWKINS: I would agree with that. It raises the question, of course, as to how a profession, ours or any other, can, acting in unison if you will, direct specific attention to an area and/or a problem. I think Dr. Sabshin demonstrated very nicely yesterday that we are not paying the attention to social factors that the problem merits. The question raised then is: How do you go about it? Maybe we will get into that.

DR. ROMANO: I would like to touch on another point. I understand fully that one certainly cannot do justice to many matters relevant to the theme of psychiatry in society within the time limitations of an exercise like this, but I was particularly impressed with the fact that in this discussion there has been no mention at all of economic factors. So I address myself principally to Dr. Rosenberg as a historian and also to Dr. Schwartz.

Many years ago Sigerist pointed out that over the centuries what happened to health, health education, health services, health-care delivery, research in health matters, etc., was a function of two variables. One was the percentage of the gross product (or, we could say, of the population concerned) that was to be devoted to health matters; and the other was what tools were available at that particular time, in terms of knowledge, skills, information, etc. If you review the 20th century very briefly, you will find that it was not only the efforts of that resolute, intrepid man, Abraham Flexner, the muckraker of our time, that brought about these remarkable changes in American medical education, but the fact that his efforts were made at a time of America's great industrial growth in the use of coal, oil, and steel. The foundations established on the profits—the Carnegie and Rockefeller and Commonwealth and others—made possible the renaissance of American medical education in the teens of this century. It was the Commonwealth Fund that gave the spark to the child guidance movement and the growth of the whole American child psychiatry program in the teens and the early twenties after World War I. Then, as I mentioned in my paper, a prodigious thing happened after World War II; our 79th Congress passed the National Mental Health Law, which for the first time made available federal moneys for research and teaching in this field. This political act of the 79th Congress was, to my mind, the most significant influence on American psychiatry, an influence that far surpassed any other. One notes the enormous growth of the American Psychiatric Association from 3,500 members in 1945–46 to more than 20,000 members at the present time, the development of a whole program of residency training, and the enrollment of a cadre of research scholars in the field, largely because of these political and economic factors.

And so I raise the question to those of you who wish to respond: Given the current urgency and the leanness of the years ahead (in terms of federal funds) that we evidently face now, will we—or, as citizens, should we—continue to turn to those agencies in which tax funds may be available to sustain research and teaching? Will there be other sources of money? For example, the movement today is to decentralize, to move from the federal to the local position, and to ask that local financing assume such responsibilities one way or another. If this shift in support is successfully made, do you believe that there will be material change in the continuing growth of the field in education and research?

DR. ROSENBERG: I would like to say that I agree wholeheartedly in terms of the significance of economic realities, if you want to call them that. Obviously, if this country had not been rich you could not have made certain kinds of decisions. As a matter of fact, the first point that I made emphasized the influence of public policies. Public policy obviously subsumes economic capacity and is always an economic decision because it relates to the allocation of resources. I think that what is in a sense tricky about psychiatry is that it is not clear how much is enough or where the investment should be made, which is a problem not only for the administration but, I think, for everyone. It is perhaps especially sensitive in psychiatry because there it is not clear where the money should be spent, or whether a given number of dollars above what is being spent would do any good.

Now the question of local funding versus national is important, I think, because it involves a question of values. National decisions have come to be defined in terms of our scientific bureaucracy. There are certain priorities. There will be a certain amount of basic research and there will be peer review. We can hope that certain standards and criteria will be met. If you turn the money over to the locality, even if the same absolute amount of money is spent, decisions as to how it will be spent are made on a local basis, and I think you will get very different kinds of decisions, ones that may be dysfunctional in terms of ultimate intellectual development within the field. I share your concern, but I simply do not know what is going to happen.

DR. SCHWARTZ: I would like to take the opportunity of using Dr. Romano's remarks to try to clarify my position. You see, there are two issues. One is a conceptual issue and the other is an action issue. What I was trying to propose is that on the conceptual issue you take what I call a "concept of context" view.

Psychiatry has progressed from looking within the individual to examining what happens between one individual and another, and then to studying the whole family system. Why do you stop with the family as the ultimate context to be viewed? I am suggesting that you move beyond that. Families are, after all, in a societal context much as the individual is in the context of the family. So that is the first problem: How do we conceptualize these different levels of complexity and perspective into some kind of coherent, sensible framework so that we can understand what brings a person to the distressed state in which he needs a psychiatrist? The second issue is: When you have gotten some handle on the conceptual problem, at what points do you intervene, and how do you do it? Again, you confine yourself to the individual and then move on to the group or the family. Why do you stop there? I presume that is the most effective way to conduct your treatment. Or is it for political purposes? Or do other kinds of considerations now getting into the picture (or in the picture all along) make it difficult or impossible to move beyond the family into society?

DR. DAIN: As a historian I have been interested in these questions for a long time. Certain considerations seem rather glaringly absent in this discussion. There seems to be no consideration of the fact that there are interests involved: the discussion goes on as if it were all consensus. It would appear that everyone's desires, needs, and hopes are all the same, and all that one has to do is to find out what is needed, tell people about it, and the need will be met! I know of no society that has ever operated on that basis. Surely one should not be surprised if psychiatrists shy away from areas very dangerous to them. Let us say they bring up economic matters, their need for funds and resources. Is it not obvious how much more difficult it would be today if psychiatrists entered into the political arena directly? It seems to me glaringly obvious that this administration or any other would consider them political opponents, not just physicians expressing scientifically determined needs and desires. The recognition of this necessarily sets limits, and I think this is partly why psychiatrists stop with the family today. If you look at the whole history of the way psychiatrists have operated—and not only psychiatrists but any other scientific or professional group—you will see that all scientists have found at various times certain areas they dared not enter at the risk of finding themselves imprisoned or rejected or vilified. It does seem to me also that there has perhaps not been sufficient discussion—in spite of a certain awareness of the fact—that the problems psychiatrists face in this respect are characteristic of the society.

The institutional arrangements of this society are in very much the same state. I would suggest to you as a hypothesis that all institutions, once they reach beyond a certain size, no longer have as a primary objective to serve the interests of the people they are supposed to serve, whether they be patients, prisoners, business people, or anyone else. When they reach a certain size their tendency is to serve the interests of those who control and run them. Administrators reassess the function for which such an institution was presumably established, and they get their rewards. Hospital superintendents received their rewards in the late 19th century for running cheap, inexpensive institutions which did not "make waves." This was the function of these men, and they were lauded when the institution was very large and therefore presumably economical. The patients did not disturb anyone. Nobody heard from the administrators and this silence was consistent with their role. It was not necessarily the role they wanted, but it was the one they were eventually forced into, partly because of their own prejudice against the kinds of patients they dealt with—class prejudice, racial prejudice, and prejudice against immigrants—and partly because of a lack of funds, in a whole complex of situations.

It does seem to me that any analysis which remains completely on the level of consensus is inadequate. Certainly it would be utterly inadequate to deal with your patients on that basis—if you failed to recognize that they had conflicts—real ones, not make-believe ones—between their needs and those of other people, and so forth. It seems to me that this is the question that has to be brought out into the open. If you decide, as you obviously have—and I cannot say that I blame you—that there are certain areas that you are very chary of, very sensitive about entering, at least be aware of this and admit it, and acknowledge the reasons why this is so.

I would make one other point. I am not convinced, at least as I study the history of psychiatry, that it is really quite fair to expect psychiatrists to enter the fray as revolutionaries, radicals, reformers, or what have you. The fact is that the type of person who goes into medicine or psychiatry is not necessarily the type of person who becomes a reformer. There were periods of time when psychiatrists were reformers and engaged in revolutionary movements, participated actively in all sorts of reforms. Benjamin Rush is an example. When the time is ripe and that is where people are going, you may expect some psychiatrists at least to go along. But there are times when society tends to be conservative and its institutions are powerful and large; then psychiatrists attempting reform have a lot to lose. The Communist party of France did not support the revolt against DeGaulle, after all. Such caution is very common. Therefore I think that perhaps one tends to put too much onus on psychiatrists; there are complaints when they seem to play the role of God and try to control the whole world. Do not reject them, then, because in certain instances they *do not* play the role of God and try to control the world. You cannot have it both ways!

Contributors

D. Wilfred Abse, m.d.—Professor of Psychiatry, School of Medicine, University of Virginia.

David L. Bazelon, ll.d.—Chief Judge of the U.S. Court of Appeals for the District of Columbia; Clinical Professor of Psychiatry (sociolegal aspects), George Washington University; Lecturer in Psychiatry, The Johns Hopkins University School of Medicine.

Norman Dain, ph.d.—Professor of History, Rutgers University; Research Associate, Payne Whitney Psychiatric Clinic, Cornell University.

Robert D. Gardner, m.d.—Psychiatrist-Director, Central Virginia Mental Health Services, Lynchburg, Virginia.

Roy R. Grinker, Sr., m.d.—Director, Institute for Psychosomatic and Psychiatric Research; Chairman of the Department of Psychiatry, Michael Reese Hospital, Chicago; Professor of Psychiatry, University of Chicago.

David R. Hawkins, m.d.—Professor and Chairman of the Department of Psychiatry, School of Medicine, University of Virginia.

Seymour S. Kety, m.d.—Professor of Psychiatry, Harvard Medical School; Director of the Psychiatric Research Laboratories, Massachusetts General Hospital, Boston.

Lawrence C. Kolb, m.d.—Professor and Chairman of the Department of Psychiatry, College of Physicians and Surgeons, Columbia University; Director, New York State Psychiatric Institute; Director of the Psychiatric Service, The Presbyterian Hospital, New York.

Morton Kramer, sc.d.—Chief, Biometry Branch, OPPE, National Institute of Mental Health; Alcohol, Drug Abuse and Mental Health Administration.

George Kriegman, m.d.—Clinical Professor of Psychiatry, Medical College of Virginia, Virginia Commonwealth University.

James L. Mathis, m.d.—Professor and Chairman of the Department of Psychiatry, Medical College of Virginia, Virginia Commonwealth University.

John Romano, m.d.—Distinguished University Professor of Psychiatry, University of Rochester School of Medicine and Dentistry.

Charles E. Rosenberg, ph.d.—Professor of History, University of

Pennsylvania; Member, History of Life Sciences Study Section, National Institute of Health.

MELVIN SABSHIN, M.D.—Former Professor and Chairman of the Department of Psychiatry, Abraham Lincoln School of Medicine and the University of Illinois College of Medicine; Medical Director, American Psychiatric Association.

MORRIS S. SCHWARTZ, PH.D.—Mortimer Gryzmish Professor in Human Relations and Chairman of the Department of Sociology, Brandeis University.

JOHN P. SPIEGEL, M.D.—Director of the Lemberg Center for the Study of Violence and Professor of Social Psychiatry, Brandeis University; President of the American Psychiatric Association.

Indexes

Subject Index

Index of Names